Curriculum Planning in Nursing Education:
Practical Applications

Curriculum Planning in Nursing Education: Practical Applications

Edited by

Stella Pendleton
MA (Ed), BH Hons (Soc and Ed), RGN, RSCN,
RM, MTD, Dip Nursing

and

Alan Myles
MA (Ed), Dip Ed, RGN, RNT

Edward Arnold
A division of Hodder & Stoughton
LONDON NEW YORK MELBOURNE AUCKLAND

© 1991 Stella Pendleton and Alan Myles

First published in Great Britain 1991

British Library Cataloguing in Publication Data

Pendleton, Stella
 Curriculum planning in nursing education.
 1. Nurses. Professional education. Curriculum Planning
 I. Title   II. Myles, Alan
 610.7307

  ISBN 0–340–51839–1

Whilst the advice and information in this book is believed to be true and accurate at the date of going to press, neither the author nor the publisher can accept any legal responsibility or liability for any errors or omissions that may be made.

Typeset in 10/11 pt Times Lasercomp
Printed and bound in Great Britain for Edward Arnold, a division of Hodder and Stoughton Limited, Mill Road, Dunton Green, Sevenoaks, Kent TN13 2YA by Biddles Limited, Guildford and King's Lynn

Foreword

This text which shows an essentially practical approach to curriculum planning is one that should be welcomed by all involved in the education of nurses, midwives and health visitors. It could also be a valuable text for those working with a wide range of students in health care.

The various authors demonstrate by their contributions the considerable progress that has been made in education. They display the developments in an imaginative and enthusiastic way while never losing sight of the fact that nursing is an essentially practice-based profession.

While there is a focus on curriculum planning for those Schools and Colleges that will be taking part in the educational reform set out in Project 2000: A New Preparation for Practice (United Kingdom Central Council for Nursing, Midwifery and Health Visiting), this should not be seen to be limiting. It is, or could be, equally applicable to staff of Schools and Colleges offering a range of other programmes. Additionally, it is important to point out that while reference is made to guidelines and papers issued by the English National Board for Nursing, Midwifery and Health Visiting, this is because, at the time of going to press, England is the only country implementing the proposals of 'Project 2000'. Although readers throughout the rest of the United Kingdom will need to await guidance from their own National Board, the principles set out should be equally applicable. It could also be regarded as a textbook that would be valuable to educators involved in health care in other countries.

While the authors have attempted to produce a book that is usable by a wide range of educationalists it is not a book for the complacent. It challenges many theories beloved by traditional educationalists but it is not destructive in its approach but constructive and should stimulate debate and discussion which will be helpful to the development of nursing education in its quest to improve the care of patients and clients.

Margaret D. Green
Deputy General Secretary/Director of Education
Royal College of Nursing

Contents

List of contributors

Jacqueline A Bryan   BSc, SRN, Dip N (Lond), Dip N Ed
Nurse Teacher, Cambridge and Huntingdon Department of Nurse Education

Anne Casey   RSCN, RGN, Dip N, Dip N Ed
Nurse Teacher, Charles West School of Nursing, Great Ormond Street, London

Sally Glen   MA, Dip Ed (Lond), RGN, RSCN, Dip N (Lond), RNT
Lecturer in Nursing Education, Institute of Education, University of London and Parkside and Harrow College of Nursing

Valerie Lattimer   RGN, Dip N (Lond), Dip N Ed
Senior Tutor, Department of Continuing Professional Education, Southampton University College of Nursing and Midwifery

Terry Maunder   BA (Hons), RMN, RNT
Nurse Tutor, Continuing Education, St Bartholomew's College of Nursing and Midwifery, London

Alan Myles   MA (Ed), Dip Ed (Lond), RGN, RNT
Principal Lecturer, Education Studies, Institute of Advanced Nursing Education, Royal College of Nursing, London

Stella Pendleton   MA (Ed), B Hum (Hons), Dip N (Lond), RGN, RSCN, RM, MTD
Principal Lecturer, Curriculum Research and Development, Institute of Advanced Nursing Education, Royal College of Nursing, London

Linda Smith   RGN, Dip N, Dip N Ed
Lecturer Practitioner in Nursing Studies, Queen Charlotte's College of Health Care Studies, London

Keiron Spires   BA, RGN, RSCN, Clinical Teachers Cert
Nurse Teacher, Computer Services, Charles West School of Nursing, Great Ormond Street, London

The Editors

Stella Pendleton   MA (Ed), B Hum (Hons), Dip N (Lond), RGN, RSCN, RM, MTD
Principal Lecturer, Curriculum Research and Development, Institute of Advanced Nursing Education, Royal College of Nursing, London

Alan Myles   MA (Ed), Dip Ed (Lond), RGN, RNT
Principal Lecturer, Education Studies, Institute of Advanced Nursing Education, Royal College of Nursing, London

Acknowledgements

Sincere thanks are extended to all the contributors for their hard work and co-operation in the preparation of this book, to Miss Moya Jolley for her inspiration, and to Miss Margaret Green for writing the Foreword. Grateful appreciation is due to staff of the Royal College of Nursing Library: to Mrs Amanda Watson for her unflagging zeal in checking and preparing the references, and to Miss Helen Thomas and Mr Tony Shepherd for their support. Thanks are also extended to the following publishers who gave permission to use copyright material in the book: to Croom Helm for permission to reproduce adaptations of Miles' 'Experiential Learning Cycle' and Beattie's Fourfold Curriculum, both taken from Allan, P. and Jolley, M. (Eds) (1987) *The Curriculum in Nursing Education*; to Slack Incorporated for permission to use an extract from Lantz, J.M. and Meyers, G D. (1986) 'Critical thinking through writing: using personification to teach pharmacodynamics', *Journal of Nursing Education*, **25(2)**, Feb. 64–6; to the Gower Publishing Group for permission to use the Cave Exercise from Woodcock, M. and Francis, D. (1982) *Activities for Self-Development: A Companion Volume of the 'Unblocked Manager'*; and to Ned Flanders for permission to reproduce his Interaction Analysis. Finally, warm appreciation is due to the Reverend Mervyn Pendleton for his invaluable help in the preparation of the manuscript, and to Miss Nancy Loffler of Edward Arnold for her patience and encouragement.

Introduction
Stella Pendleton

Nurse educators have a key role in facilitating the professional and personal development of students and thereby in maintaining and improving standards of patient and client care. The 1990s will see far reaching changes in nursing education in the United Kingdom and this book is offered in the belief that, in fulfilling their role, nurse educators need curriculum planning skills based on sound theoretical principles. For educational theory can contribute to thoughtful and defensible curriculum decision-making and can guide and illuminate practice. Theory, however, has its limitations; for as Schwab (1969) points out, it deals with the general, the abstract and the ideal, whereas the curriculum 'will be brought to bear not in some archetypal classroom but in a particular locus in time and space with smells, shadows, seats, and conditions outside its walls which may have much to do with what is achieved inside'. And so, too, in nursing education, the curriculum is enacted in the realm of the particular: with particular students and a particular teacher, in a specific classroom with its impossible-to-write-upon chalkboard and the overhead projector that obstinately refuses to focus; with particular clinical staff struggling in difficult circumstances to maintain standards and provide a good service for a unique community. Educational theory, therefore, may need to be adapted to suit particular settings. In the same way, while this book offers suggestions as to how theory can be used in practice, it is likely that some modifications may be needed to suit individual, unique educational contexts. This is an important point, because although several chapters focus particularly on Project 2000 (United Kingdom Central Council for Nursing, Midwifery and Health Visiting, 1986), nevertheless the ideas and principles put forward have wider applications.

The first chapter of the book serves as an introduction and Stella Pendleton provides a broad overview of key curricular elements within a dialectical framework. She includes discussion of educational philosophies, curriculum planning models, the selection and organisation of content and learning experiences, assessment, evaluation and innovation. In Chapter 2 the dialectical approach is taken up by Sally Glen in the context of planning what is, perhaps, the most difficult area of a nursing curriculum: the ethics component. She includes worked examples showing how a dialectical approach can assist in selecting strategies for teaching ethics, and her chapter ends with suggestions for assessing this part of a Common Foundation Programme. Sally Glen argues that situational analysis (Skilbeck, 1984) forms a useful part of the planning process, and the theme of curriculum planning models recurs in Chapter 3 in which Anne Casey discusses how Lawton's (1983) cultural analysis model was used in conjunction with a nursing model to plan a curriculum for part 8 (Sick Children) of the professional register. In Chapter 4 Terry Maunder suggests that sociological theory can enhance a nurse's understanding of a nursing model and better equip him or her to meet the needs of patients. He outlines some sociological content areas which could form part of a Common Foundation Programme for a Project 2000 course, and includes some worked examples to show how sociology can be taught to nurses in interesting and stimulating ways.

Teaching methods are a key concern of Jacqueline Bryan who, in Chapter 5, chooses an area of the curriculum which she believes poses a particular challenge for teachers wishing to adopt a student-centred approach. Drawing on Brunerian theory she suggests how learning the nursing care of patients with haematological disorders can be made a challenging and satisfying experience for students. She provides worked examples of a range of teaching methods and includes discussion of suitable assessment strategies. Linda Smith is also concerned to provide meaningful learning experiences for students and in Chapter 6 she argues strongly for changes in the curriculum so that nurses are helped to develop more positive attitudes towards caring for elderly people. She gives a number of suggestions as to how the development of such attitudes could be facilitated and the activities described would be suitable for pre- and post-registration students.

In Chapter 7 Alan Myles examines an area of nursing education which is likely to expand in the 1990s. Drawing on the tenets of andragogy and the concept of social need he explores the nature of independent study and then discusses the principles and practice of open/distance learning, contract learning and projects as examples of independent study. He pays particular attention to the issues involved in assessing projects and proposes a list of criteria to improve the validity and reliability of marking schemes. Valerie Lattimer tackles a curriculum element which is also likely to become increasingly important in the future: the evaluation of teaching effectiveness. In Chapter 8 she discusses evaluation by self, peers and students and proposes a number of practical suggestions to help teachers who wish to explore ways of improving the quality of their teaching. Information Technology is another potential growth area in nursing education and in Chapter 9 Keiron Spires draws on change theory to suggest how this innovation could be introduced into a curriculum. In the final chapter, Stella Pendleton examines curriculum decision-making as a whole. She discusses the nature of curriculum problems and includes suggestions about the composition and functioning of curriculum development groups.

Readers will find no uniformity of style or presentation in these chapters, and the proportion of theory and practical application differs from author to author. It is hoped that this diversity will add to the interest of the book and that teachers at all levels of experience will find it provides useful insights. Those who already have varying degrees of theoretical knowledge should discover new ways of applying it, while those with plenty of practical experience but little theoretical knowledge may be stimulated to explore this more deeply. Hopefully, too, readers will *enjoy* this book! Eisner (1985) notes the 'sober, humorless quality of so much of the writing in the field of curriculum', and he argues that the 'tendency toward what is believed to be scientific language has resulted in an emotionally eviscerated form of expression; any sense of the poetic or the passionate must be excised. Instead, the aspiration is to be value-neutral and technical ... . Cool, dispassionate objectivity has resulted in sterile, mechanistic language devoid of the playfulness and artistry that are so essential to teaching and learning'. Readers will find in this book snatches of playfulness, humour and passion, and possibly areas with which they disagree. Hopefully they will gain ideas for reflection and suggestions which can be tried out, tested and refined in practice.

Eisner, E.W. (1985). *The Educational Imagination: On the Design and Evaluation of School Programs*. Second edition. Macmillan, New York.

Lawton, D. (1983). *Curriculum Studies and Educational Planning*. Hodder & Stoughton, London.

Schwab, J.J. (1969). The practical: a language for curriculum. *School Review*, **78**, Nov., 1–23.

Skilbeck, M. (1984). *School-based Curriculum Development*. Harper and Row, London.

United Kingdom Central Council for Nursing, Midwifery and Health Visiting (1986) *Project 2000: A New Preparation for Practice*. UKCC, London.

1 Curriculum planning in nursing education: towards the year 2000

Stella Pendleton

Imagine a rather unusual curriculum development group meeting. The panelled oak walls are hung with still portraits of venerable toads, some wearing gowns and mortarboards, who look down silently on the assembled company. But there is nothing still and silent about the present incumbent of Toad Hall. Canary yellow caravans, boats, and red motor cars are all forgotten in the excitement of the Water-Rat's suggestion that part of Toad Hall should be converted into a school for the animals of the neighbourhood. We join the group as they begin to explore the purposes of the education they plan to offer.

'I think it's very important that animals should have the chance to learn skills like counting and cooking and,' Mole hesitates, 'spring cleaning. Practical things that will be useful.' 'I see your point, Moly,' the Rat says tolerantly, 'but should education *really* be concerned with skills and the world of work? Aren't there some things that are worth learning just because they're valuable in themselves? Things like poetry and music and the history of our river banks and woods?'

Toad can contain himself no longer. 'The history of the illustrious House of Toad is essential!' he exclaims. 'But animals must be free to grow and develop; to learn the things that interest them; to explore, to travel the open road of knowledge, turning down exciting paths when distant vistas beckon!'

Toad carries on in a similar vein for several minutes while Badger, who has not yet spoken, waits for the excited animal to stop for a breath.

'You know,' Badger remarks at last, 'we seem to be missing something.' He pauses, taking a sip of Toad's elderberry wine, before continuing thoughtfully. 'I should like to think that we could help to build a better world through education. A world where no creature ever died of hunger or thirst or suffered from preventable illness, and where everyone had a warm home.'

Even Toad falls silent at the enormity of the task.

'These are big things,' the Rat says at last.

'Yes,' replies the Badger, 'but perhaps we can start in a very limited way, here, in our own school, by our own river banks and in our own woods and fields.'

The above discussion takes us to some of the fundamental purposes of education and to the very heart of the curriculum planning process. This chapter therefore begins by considering the four ideologies represented by Mole, Rat, Toad and Badger, in relation to nursing education. Links will be made with Beattie's (1987) Fourfold Curriculum and a fourfold approach will be used to analyse and clarify some curriculum planning models. Following this, suggestions will be made as to how the same approach can help in the formulation of a philosophy in nursing education. A four-dimensional model of the curriculum will then be proposed and applied to the planning of a Common Foundation Programme for Project 2000 (United Kingdom Central Council for Nursing, Midwifery and Health Visiting, 1986). The last part of the chapter suggests how the same model can help in the planning of assessment schemes, and in curriculum evaluation. A discussion of curriculum innovation ends the chapter.

Four educational ideologies

The contrasting beliefs expressed in the opening scenario represent different ideologies about the whole enterprise of education. 'Ideologies' is being used here in one of the senses described by Scrimshaw (1983), i.e. as 'sets of values and beliefs which are, on occasion, given fairly clear and systematic expression in documents, speeches, and so on. In these terms, they are simply like philosophies.'

Instrumentalism

Mole's ideology is related to the needs of society for a skilled workforce. Thus, as Marson (1980) argues, the content and process of education are seen mainly as means to social and economic ends, and there is an emphasis on the 'relevance and utility aspects of knowledge' (cited by Scrimshaw, 1983). For the instrumentalist, the content and learning experiences provided for students would therefore be justified on extrinsic grounds (for example, the acquisition of sound practical skills to provide a safe public service) rather than intrinsic grounds such as the value of the content and learning experiences *in themselves*. All of this may suggest that instrumentalists are concerned with 'training' rather than 'education'. However, Scrimshaw (1983) distinguishes between 'traditional' and 'adaptive' instrumentalism. The former is associated with an apprenticeship system which involves instruction in defined vocational skills, practical problem-solving and the inculcation of good work habits. This version of instrumentalism seems to relate to 'training' and 'instruction' which Stenhouse (1975) suggests are two of the processes comprising 'education'. Training is 'concerned with the acquisition of skills, and successful training results in capacity in performance.... Instruction is concerned with the learning of information and successful instruction results in retention' (Stenhouse, 1975).

The second version of instrumentalism seems to go beyond training and instruction. Scrimshaw (1983) suggests that as technical training becomes more complex, specific vocational skills may not be adequate to meet societal needs and the acquisition of more general skills and capacities becomes necessary. Thus adaptive instrumentalists emphasise the active learning of life skills, through group work and guided discussion, as well as the acquisition of practical problem-solving skills. Such an approach might suggest that the teacher is at times a guide as well as an instructor. This version of instrumentalism would seem to encompass not only training and instruction but also 'initiation', which Stenhouse (1975) sees as being concerned with 'familiarization with social values and norms'. Successful initiation, he argues, 'leads to a capacity to interpret the social environment and to anticipate the reaction to one's own actions'. The fourth process described by Stenhouse (1975) as comprising 'education' is 'induction' and this is for him the key factor in a truly educative process. 'Induction stands for introduction into the thought systems – the knowledge – of the culture and successful induction results in understanding as evidenced by the capacity to grasp and make for oneself relationships and judgements' (Stenhouse, 1975).

The issues raised here are far from theoretical when viewed in the light of the National Council for Vocational Qualifications (NCVQ) (1987) Framework, and the preparation of nurses and health care assistants (support workers). The NCVQ was set up by the Government in 1986 and NCVQ (n.d.) state the purposes and aims of the new framework. The opening paragraph of the foreword is interesting in the light of the foregoing discussion of instrumentalism as an ideology:

'The last few years have seen a tremendous expansion in training provision in this country, which will not only help to improve the competence of our workforce but will also increase the competitiveness of our industry. This has led to calls by many for a more coherent and understandable system of vocational qualifications.'

NCVQ (1987) define a 'vocational qualification' as

'a statement of competence – skills, knowledge, understanding and ability in application – needed to facilitate entry into, or progression in employment and/or further education and training, which incorporates assessment to specified standards of: skills; relevant knowledge and understanding; the ability to use skills and apply knowledge and understanding to the performance of work related activities.'

At the time of going to print four levels of qualifications have been described and further work is under way to include the professions in the higher levels of the NCVQ framework. Department of Health (1990) state that 'It will be for the NCVQ to determine at what levels within that framework the qualifications will be awarded, but work is proceeding on the hypothesis that most HCA (Health Care Assistant) qualifications will be at levels 2 and 3.' Level 3 qualifications will indicate 'ability to perform a broad range of work-related activities, including many that are complex, difficult and non-routine, appropriate to sustaining regular processes and outputs, to specified standards' (NCVQ, 1987).

Returning to Stenhouse's (1975) discussion about the importance of education, it could be argued that health care assistants will be involved in all four processes including induction, since they are required to have understanding and at level 3 will be coping with 'non-routine activities'. In other words, health care assistants, like the new Project 2000 practitioners, could be said to be 'educated'. This is a crucial issue because of the dangers associated with blurring of role boundaries between the two groups. Role confusion and possible exploitation of health care assistants could ensue, neither of which is likely to enhance patient/client care. The problems of role confusion are even more relevant when considering the role of health care assistants and enrolled nurses, but in the interest of brevity this discussion will focus on the preparation of Project 2000 practitioners.

It was suggested above that since health care assistants are required to show evidence of 'understanding' and some flexibility, they could be said to be educated. However, it is relevant to note that though the activities at NCVQ (1987) level 3 may include those that are 'non-routine', nevertheless they sustain 'regular processes and outputs'. It would seem that a limited form of flexibility is involved and the same also could be said to apply to the 'understanding' required. Health care assistants will certainly need to have an understanding of the rationale for their activities but this arguably falls short of Stenhouse's (1975) conception of knowledge which can 'sustain creative thought and provide frameworks for judgement'.

The issue of what is involved in 'education' is also of great significance as partnerships are formed between schools/colleges of nursing and higher education institutions, and as joint validations are sought from professional and academic bodies. This exploration of the nature of education will therefore be continued in the light of the other three ideologies, beginning with liberal humanism.

Liberal humanism

Liberal humanism differs from instrumentalism in the way decisions about content and learning experiences in the curriculum are justified. For the instrumentalist decisions are justified on extrinsic grounds such as usefulness to the needs of society, whereas for the liberal humanist the grounds relate to the intrinsic worthwhileness of the curricular content and activities. In other words, such content and activities are seen as being worthwhile *in themselves*. Kelly (1986) asserts that this approach has its roots in a rationalist view of knowledge which dates back to Plato and embodies the assumption that knowledge has an objective reality independent of the shifting and unreliable experience of the senses. Such experience cannot be the source of knowledge and yet some degree of certainty must be possible with regard to human knowledge. The only source of knowledge must therefore be the rational mind. The legacy of this view of knowledge is still evident and can be identified in the words of educational philosophers such as Peters (1966) and Hirst (1974). Thus Hirst (1974) sees education as being 'concerned directly with the development of the mind in rational knowledge ...' and he compares his view with the original Greek concept which saw a liberal education as 'freeing of the mind to achieve its own good in knowledge'. Hirst (1974) believes knowledge can be logically classified into distinct but related forms, each having its own concepts, and criteria of truth or validity, and each involving 'the making of a distinctive form of reasoned judgement ...'. As Stenhouse (1975) points out, Hirst does not claim absolute objectivity for knowledge, and Hirst (1974) himself explicitly dissociates himself from Plato's epistemology. He recognises that knowledge can change but he argues that concepts such as space and causality, for example, have stability, generality, and a relatively timeless nature.

Hirst and Peters (1970) describe seven forms of knowledge, for example, the physical sciences, 'awareness and understanding of our own and other people's minds' and moral judgement and awareness. These forms of knowledge should form the basis of all pupils' education, since to deprive a child of initiation into any of these forms would limit his development and his ability to achieve the good life. *Classical* humanists, it should be noted in passing, argue that some pupils should study intellectual disciplines while others should be engaged in practical and aesthetic areas (Scrimshaw, 1983). However, liberal humanists would want all children to be initiated into certain areas of knowledge in the curriculum, either because of their intrinsic value (Rat and his poetry in the opening scenario!) or because they promote the development of rational thought. The word 'initiated' is important since it implies that the teacher possesses expert knowledge which is passed on to pupils. This does not necessarily mean that pupils are *uncritical* recipients, and it is worth noting that Peters (1966) regards 'teaching' as involving 'the passing on of knowledge, skills, or modes of conduct in such a way that the learner is brought to understand and evaluate the underlying rationale for what is presented to him'. The phrases 'passing on' and 'presented to him' suggest a fairly teacher-centred approach, but even so, the notion of 'passive learners' applies to *classical*, rather than liberal humanism. It is significant that Hirst (1974) does not imply that curriculum activities should be determined only by teachers, without any changes being made by pupils.

In considering liberal humanism in relation to nursing education we come up against the question of justification. For the biological, physical and social sciences and the humanities certainly form an important part of the nursing curriculum, but it could be said that their inclusion is on *extrinsic* grounds, as a means, directly or indirectly, of enhancing nursing practice. However, it could be argued that studying such disciplines can also be *intrinsically* worthwhile in contributing to the personal development of the nurses. For the disciplines can enrich students' understanding of what Peters (1981) calls the 'human condition', and the study of science can be viewed not simply in instrumental terms but as 'the study of the beauty of the world' (Weil, 1952). Moreover, studying the disciplines can help further the development of those intellectual virtues described by Peters (1981) as 'consistency, hatred of irrelevance, clarity, precision, accuracy and a determination to look at the facts'. Much depends on the *way* academic subjects are taught. Chapter 4 of this book shows how an academic subject can be related to nursing practice and taught in ways that help students become familiar with the necessary body of knowledge through intellectually demanding and stimulating processes. The issue of intrinsic worthwhileness of content is also relevant to the question of liberal studies for nurses. It is perhaps a pity that the liberal studies component proposed in the English National Board for Nursing, Midwifery and Health Visiting (ENB) (1985) Consultation Paper does not seem to have materialised in the current proposals for future pre-registration nursing education. However, this should not preclude individual schools/colleges of nursing from taking this initiative themselves.

Liberal humanism thus stresses the knowledge content of the curriculum and the intellectual development of students. It embodies a relatively objective view of knowledge and in this respect it has something in common with instrumentalism. The objectivity of knowledge inherent in the latter ideology, however, stems from an instrumental concern to teach 'packages' of knowledge, skills and attitudes in a way that tends to stress correct and safe practices rather than encouraging a more open-ended and enquiring approach to learning. By contrast, the liberal humanist's view of knowledge is related to a rationalist epistemology. The two ideologies also differ, as has been shown, in the way the selection of content and learning experiences are justified, instrumentalism basing decisions on extrinsic factors and liberal humanism on intrinsic factors. A third ideology, progressivism, has nothing in common with instrumentalism and only a little more in common with liberal humanism.

Progressivism

Progressivism is rooted in seventeenth century empiricism, a view of knowledge which emerged in opposition to that of the rationalists (Kelly, 1986). According to the empiricist the only real source of knowledge is sense experience, which by its nature tends to be somewhat unreliable. Thus knowledge, far from having a relatively stable, timeless quality, is seen as tentative and hypothetical. Indeed, as Blenkin and Kelly (1987) point out, for an extreme empiricist such as Hume, the possibility of knowing anything with a degree of certainty was open to question. This new challenge to rationalism had considerable implications for educational practice. For if knowledge is so tentative then it is difficult to have very definite ideas as to what kinds of knowledge should be included in the curriculum. Moreover, if the only real source of knowledge is sense experience, then the personal experience of each individual becomes very important in the educational process. Thus Rousseau, who could be called the founder of progressivism, emphasised the promotion of natural growth in the child and active learning from experience, rather than the imposition of knowledge. His advice was: 'Give your scholar no verbal lessons, he should be taught by experience alone. . . . Put the problems before him and let him solve them himself. Let him know nothing because you have told him, but because he has learnt it for himself. Let him not be taught science, let him discover it' (cited by Blenkin and Kelly, 1987).

The above quotations bring together a number of concepts that have a very modern ring! Learning from experience, discovery learning and problem-solving were all being advocated in 1762 (the year Rousseau's *Emile* was published) and they constituted a major challenge to the rationalist view of education which had held sway since Plato's time. However, empiricism, especially in its extreme form, was and is problematic, particularly in the realm of knowledge relating to values. For as Kelly (1986) points out, empiricism provides no grounds for any certainty or assurance in the area of values.

It was this dilemma, posed by the epistemologies of rationalism and empiricism, that Dewey's pragmatism sought to reconcile (Kelly, 1986). Dewey (1916) draws the distinction between objective and impersonal *knowledge* and subjective and personal *thinking*. Knowledge is that which is settled and established, and which we assume without question at a given time. By contrast, thinking starts from doubt or uncertainty. 'It marks an inquiring, hunting, searching attitude, instead of one of mastery and possession. Through its critical process true knowledge is revised and extended, and our convictions as to the state of things reorganized' (Dewey, 1916). The scientific experimental method is the means of getting knowledge and ensuring it *is* knowledge and not opinion. Educative experiences involve thinking. This means that a pupil reflects on genuine problems which have arisen out of activities which interest him. He uses information and observation to deal with problems, formulating possible solutions and testing ideas by application so as to clarify their meaning and discover for himself their validity (Dewey, 1916). For Dewey education is a lifelong process of growth not a means to an extrinsic end.

The progressivist ideology thus embodies an open view of knowledge and an emphasis on the processes of growth and development in the learner rather than on content to be acquired. In the opening extract Toad represents a progressive ideology, but his own tendency to flit from interest to interest (from boats to the yellow caravan to the red motor car) would not accurately represent the views of those educationalists such as Kelly (1989) whose thinking builds upon the progressivist inheritance. Thus Kelly (1989) argues that 'those activities that are intrinsically valuable are those that the children do actually value in themselves and that, as a result, a curriculum can be truly described as educational only if its content consists of those things that children value and *through the pursuit of which their development will be promoted*' (my italics). So the teacher is there as a facilitator to help learners follow and deepen their interests and, in so doing, to further their development. 'Development' for Kelly (1989) includes moral, social, affective and cognitive dimensions. Thinking related to forms of understanding such as history and science are included but it is the thinking *processes* which are important rather than the knowledge-content.

Progressivists and liberal humanists differ, then, in their view of knowledge and also on the grounds upon which curricular decisions are made. In each case justification is on grounds of 'intrinsic worthwhileness' but this concept is interpreted differently. Liberal humanists relate 'intrinsic worthwhileness' to the particular content *in itself* or the intellectual processes *in themselves*. Intrinsic worthwhileness in this instance has an objective quality. Progressivists, however, stress that 'intrinsic worthwhileness' depends on the learner's response, on whether or not the experience is worthwhile for him or her. Here 'intrinsic worthwhileness' has a personal quality.

In considering the relevance of progressivism to nursing education, the question of justification emerges immediately, as it did with liberal humanism. For nursing education is centrally concerned with the promotion of high quality patient/client care and content and learning experiences are primarily selected with this in mind. However, Dewey (1916) makes the distinction between 'training *for* occupations' and 'training *through* occupations' (this includes professional occupations). He argues that the 'only sufficient preparation for later responsibilities comes by making the most of immediately present life ...', and that

'Education *through* occupations ... combines within itself more of the factors conducive to learning than any other method. It calls instincts and habits into play; it is a foe to passive receptivity'. This suggests that every effort should be made to try and ensure that learning experiences in nursing education are intrinsically worthwhile in the progressivist sense already described. Involving students in planning decisions, affording them the maximum choice possible, and making time available for discussion and reflection about their experiences are some of the ways learning can become intrinsically worthwhile. In Chapter 6 suggestions are made as to how teaching methods can be selected to help students care sensitively for elderly people and at the same time facilitate the personal development of students. The whole concept of active student involvement in the learning process and the facilitation of self-directed learning help to ensure that education is indeed a lifelong process. It is interesting, also, to note that in the UKCC's (1988) proposals for future pre-registration nursing education it is recognised that the development of processes such as problem-solving, critical thinking and analysis, are important, together with more affective processes such as coping with feelings and emotions.

Progressivism thus has much to offer nursing education and serves to remind us of the importance of facilitating the personal development of students. It has a good deal in common with Knowles' (1978) theory of andragogy and Rogers' (1983) view of education. However, let us turn now to a fourth ideology – reconstructionism – which emphasises the role of education in bringing about change in society.

Reconstructionism

Dewey was influential not only in the development of progressivism but also of reconstructionism. The view of 'education as growth' is linked with the idea that education is a process of reorganising or reconstructing experience. This reorganisation makes experience more meaningful and increases a person's control over the direction of future experiences. The *individual* development of future citizens through restructuring of experiences could, Dewey (1916) suggested, result in the improvement of society, so that 'every person shall be occupied in something which makes the lives of others better worth living, and which accordingly makes the ties which bind persons together more perceptible ...' Skilbeck (1982a) suggests that reconstructionists emphasise a core curriculum in which current societal norms and practices are 'analysed, criticized and reconstructed according to rationalistic, democratic, communitarian values ...'. As with progressivism there is a focus on active, group learning processes such as projects and problem-solving activities.

There are problems with reconstructionism as an ideology, not least because of its utopianism. It is possible, though, to adopt a piecemeal approach to social change, such as that advocated by Badger at the beginning of this chapter. However, there must also be a concern about indoctrination. The teaching methods suggest an open view of knowledge but a teacher could, nevertheless, use his or her authority to indoctrinate students. The best safeguard would seem to be to discuss the reconstructionist ideology openly so that students could make up their own minds about their response to it. Turning now to nursing education, the question to consider is whether this ideology has any relevance. In relation to Dewey's (1916) vision of an improved society, nurses are in the happy position of helping to make 'the lives of others better worth living', but much more could be done. The key area would seem to be that of health promotion. The English National Board for Nursing, Midwifery and Health Visiting (ENB) (1989a) define 'health promotion' as 'any measure which promotes health or prevents disease', and argue that this has both a personal and public element. Thus health promotion includes not only health education about personal lifestyle but also a healthy public policy so that it is easier for consumers to make healthy choices. Already there are signs of an increasing awareness within the nursing profession about the effects of the environment on health, for example the dangers of ozone depletion, toxic waste and air pollution (Carlisle, 1989; Feinmann, 1989; Walsh, 1989). Then there are more specific health problems such as those associated with home-lessness and child poverty. It is interesting to note in this respect that the Royal College of Nursing of the United Kingdom (RCN) (1989) *Standards of Care for Health Visiting* suggests that health visitors should 'actively contribute to the development and determination, at all levels, of social policy and social change to promote health'. With a growing emphasis on community care there will, however, be increasing opportunities for nurses to be involved in shaping public health policies and working with client groups. As UKKC (1985) pointed out

'Reorientation towards the community ... means reorientation of many traditions in nursing. Traditionally, nursing has not been very good at empowering people, teaching patients, parents and clients, working in partnership, even though these ideas are now being emphasised.... Working with self-help groups, and with campaigning groups ... have been seen as peripheral problems or issues only for the few specialisms, not issues for the broad mass within nursing.'

(UKCC, 1985)

These issues are most important and demand of educators more than a raising of awareness in students. They imply, for example, that teachers should help students acquire the necessary skills, in effect, to 'be political'. The emphasis on nurses becoming active politically is particularly evident in the discussions of the International Council of Nurses and the general ethos of the World Health Organisation. It was in the context of a 'Countdown 2000' conference that Virginia Henderson wrote:

'I believe that health workers, particularly nurses, are more keenly aware of human needs and human suffering than are most people. We should therefore be in the forefront of those who work for social justice, for a healthful environment, for access to adequate food, shelter and clothing, and universal opportunities for education and employment, realizing that all of these as well as preventive and curative health care are essential to the wellbeing of citizens.'

(Henderson, 1989)

The reconstructionist ideology seems most relevant to nursing education and the inclusion of social, political and economic studies in the UKCC's (1988) draft guide lines for future pre-registration courses is to be welcomed.

Four ideologies of education have been discussed and it has been suggested that all have something to offer nursing education. Instrumentalism serves as a reminder that the safe and competent performance of practical nursing skills is necessary to protect the general public, and is linked with cost-effectiveness. Currie and Maynard (1989), for example, cite handwashing and non-touch dressing techniques as two of the proven methods of controlling hospital acquired infection. Yet it can be argued that a sound academic knowledge base, well applied, is also necessary for the provision of high quality patient/client care, and this is where liberal humanism complements instrumentalism. Liberal humanism can be criticised for embodying a view of education which is too cognitive and which places too much emphasis on knowledge-content, but such content can be taught in a way that facilitates students' personal development. The key concern of progressivism is individual development and the emphasis on its affective, as well as cognitive dimensions, complements the intellectualism of liberal humanism. Moreover, progressivism stresses the value of student experience and activity in the educative process and Dewey's idea of education as a lifelong process of growth is very relevant to the concept of continuing professional education. Progressivism's concern with individual development is balanced by the reconstructionist ideology which seeks to promote the development of a better society through education. Nurses have a key role in health promotion and nurse educators have a crucial part to play in the preparation of future practitioners for this role.

These four ideologies can be seen to underpin the four design briefs described by Skilbeck (1984) which in turn have been adapted by Beattie (1987) to form his Fourfold Curriculum. In each of the four approaches the curriculum is defined differently, i.e. as: 'a schedule of basic skills', 'a map of key subjects', 'a portfolio of meaningful personal experiences' and 'an agenda of important cultural issues'. These four approaches seem to relate to instrumentalism, liberal humanism, progressivism and reconstructionism respectively, and the views of knowledge and justification for learning described by Beattie (1987) correspond to those already discussed in relation to the four ideologies. The Fourfold Curriculum will be explored in greater detail later in this chapter, but the intention now is to use the fourfold approach to analyse and clarify some curriculum planning models.

Curriculum planning models

The behavioural objectives model

This model relates to Beattie's (1987) 'schedule of basic skills' and is associated with instrumentalism. There have been various modifications of the model but since most of the criticisms apply to 'strict' versions it is helpful to consider what is implied by such versions. Sockett (1976a) suggests that the four key features are as follows:

(a) 'that education can be defined as the *process of changing behaviour* or as *changing behaviour*'
(b) 'that the ends of the curriculum, generally referred to as *objectives*, are stated in *behavioural* form'
(c) '*that such objectives are measurable*'
(d) 'that both the *content* of what is taught and the *method* by which it is taught are seen as a *means* to these behavioural, measurable objectives'

(Sockett, 1976a)

Hamilton *et al.* (1977) note the assumption in this model that 'goal consensus in education ... is a matter of clarification rather than reconciliation'. Behavioural objectives, then, refer to intended change in learner behaviour, and should be 'absolutely specific, measurable and unambiguous' (Sockett, 1976b). The emphasis in this model is on the specific end products of learning rather than the processes of learning. Product is here interpreted as referring to the student's observable and measurable *performance* as pre-specified by behavioural objectives, for example, the competent administration of an injection. However, 'product' can also refer to a *static object* produced by the student, for example, a piece of written work. Such work would only be relevant to the behavioural objectives model if it involved the demonstration of measurable 'packages of knowledge', for example, the correct dosages of drugs. An essay requiring the student to make his or her own evaluative judgements about, say, current issues in nursing would count as a 'product' in Rowntree's (1987) terms, but would not relate to the behavioural objectives model, because this model embodies a closed view of knowledge and is concerned with specific kinds of measurable end-results.

There is no shortage of literature on the debate about the behavioural objectives model, and the intention is not to explore the arguments here, though a short critique is included in Chapter 10. It is sufficient to note here that a whole nursing curriculum based on the behavioural objectives model would imply a 'training' rather than an 'education'. The model is rooted in instrumentalism and the contribution of the other three ideologies is missing. Nevertheless, as Beattie (1987) argues, behavioural objectives have a place in the nursing curriculum in the area of practical skills, and he stresses the importance of ensuring that the teaching of such skills is based on up-to-date empirical research.

The issue of objectives is, however, rather more complex than has been implied in the discussion so far. Indeed objectives can be used in such a way that none of Sockett's (1976a) four features is present. This takes us from the behavioural objectives model to a consideration of curriculum planning based on content.

Planning by specification of content

This approach to curriculum planning is associated with liberal human-ism and is what Beattie (1987) refers to as drawing up a map of key subjects. This does not necessarily involve the use of objectives but for Hirst (1974) it does. However, his view about objectives are very differ-ent from those associated with the behavioural objectives model. He regards teaching as an intentional activity and argues that teachers should therefore specify what achievements they wish pupils to reach. Hirst himself is concerned with the cognitive development of pupils through a study of all the forms of knowledge, and setting objectives is a way of making clear how his curricular decisions are being *justified*. He explicitly rejects the behavioural objectives model, suggesting that 'if the objectives are mischaracterised in strictly behavioural terms, cur-riculum planning might well get close to planning a production line'.

With regard to the organisation of the curriculum, Hirst and Peters (1970) suggest that subjects may be based on single forms of knowledge or they may draw on several different forms. They stress, though, the importance of ensuring that students grasp the particular concepts and tests for truth associated with each form of knowledge, as well as the relationship between the forms. These points are relevant when we come to consider Bruner's (1977) approach to curriculum planning. Before doing so, however, it is worth noting that the sort of disciplines and subjects which underpin and illuminate nursing practice, can be inte-grated in the nursing curriculum as themes, for example, 'Equalities and Inequalities in Health' (Beattie, 1987). Beattie (1987) also includes the arts and sciences of nursing and medicine in his list of disciplines and subjects. Turning from a planning approach which stresses the content of the curriculum and the cognitive development of students, and is associated with liberal humanism, some process models and their associated ideologies are now considered.

Planning by specification of processes

Process models of curriculum planning may at first sight appear to be associated with progressivism. Yet both Stenhouse (1975) and Bruner (1977) appear to have been influenced by ideas from the liberal humanist tradition. Thus Stenhouse (1975) accepts Peters' (1966) notion of intrinsically worthwhile knowledge, and referring to the structure of forms of knowledge and the associated concepts, procedures, standards and criteria, suggests that a curriculum can be planned, not by behavioural objectives, but by selecting content to exemplify such key concepts, procedures and so on. For example, causation is a key concept in history, experiment a key procedure in the physical sciences, and art has its own standards and criteria by which works may be evaluated. Stenhouse (1975) argues that these concepts, procedures and criteria are the 'focus of speculation, not the object of mastery'; they 'constitute a raw material for thinking.' Thus Stenhouse emphasises the *process* of learning, for example creative thinking, speculating, reflecting, rather than the *product* of learning, i.e. the students' observable and measurable performance as pre-specified by behavioural objectives. (It should be noted in passing that Stenhouse's use of the word 'process' here is different from that used by Wheeler (1967) in his 'simple curriculum process'. This refers not to a process model but to five phases which Wheeler suggests curriculum planners should work through. The first of these phases includes the selection of objectives.) Returning to Stenhouse's (1975) process model, however, it is clear that this approach suggests a more open view of knowledge than that of instrumentalism and probably more open than that usually associated with liberal humanism.

Bruner (1977) too, seems to draw on liberal humanism. He stresses the importance of teaching the underlying structure of fields of enquiry, and Chapter five provides a worked example of how a Brunerian approach can be used to teach the nursing care of patients with haematological disorders. Interestingly, Skilbeck (1984) links Bruner and Hirst in the same tradition. However, Bruner (1966) also asserts that 'structure must always be related to the status and gifts of the learner. Viewed in this way, the optimal structure of a body of knowledge is not absolute but relative'. This seems more in keeping with the progressivist tradition and it is significant that 'the pedagogical aims' for Bruner's curriculum project 'Man: A Course of Study' were related to the processes of learning rather than the content, for example 'To encourage children to reflect on their own experiences' (Hanley *et al.*, 1970; cited by Stenhouse, 1975). All this suggests that it is an oversimplification to view ideologies as ideal types, and that elements from more than one ideology can influence an individual's thought. It should be pointed out, too, that in Stenhouse's (1975) Humanities Curriculum Project the content was not based on the forms of knowledge but on controversial issues that divide people in society. His 'principles of procedure' (corresponding to Bruner's 'pedagogical aims') defined classroom processes in terms of what the teacher was to do, and the emphasis was on an open view of knowledge. Stenhouse (1975) suggests that the behavioural objectives model is appropriate for the training and instruction components of the educational process, but he argues that education 'as induction into knowledge is successful to the extent that it makes the behavioural outcomes of students unpredictable'. For induction into knowledge he advocates the process model. However, Stenhouse (1985) asserts that

'a curriculum and teaching strategy cannot be derived from definitions of content and teacher and pupil role and aim alone. Intersecting with these are educational principles or values of a more general sort: a desire that education shall socialize or shall emancipate, a conviction that access to knowledge is central to education, a belief that education involves certain values, a preference for rationality over irrationality, for sensitivity over insensitivity, for integrity of feeling over sentimentality and so forth.'

(Stenhouse, 1985)

Stenhouse (1985) argues that it is not the objectives model that is needed to bring clarity and rigour into teaching. Rather we need 'to seek profounder analyses and greater rigour within traditional approaches'.

The concept 'process' has been used several times in the above discussion and, to explore this further, the interpretation of Blenkin and Kelly (1987) will be considered. They stress that 'process' in the context of a 'process model' and 'education as process' does not denote the procedures or methods by which children acquire the knowledge someone else has predetermined they should learn. Kelly (1989) rejects the use of objectives and agrees with Stenhouse's (1975) advocacy of 'principles of procedure' in planning but argues further that 'these principles should be derived from the view that the prime concern of the educational process is with human development'. So by 'processes' Blenkin and Kelly (1987) mean 'processes of development' in 'personal, social, moral, aesthetic, emotional as well as intellectual' dimensions. Such developmental processes are the purposes of education, and these purposes are seen as procedural principles guiding the teacher's practice throughout (Kelly, 1989). So critical thinking, for example, is a developmental process, and developing a student's skills in this area is both a purpose of education and a procedural principle.

However, the process model has been criticised and Skilbeck (1984) argues against specifying teacher activity in terms of principles of procedure. He suggests that if, for example, a speculative stance is an important feature and outcome of education then an objective should be set, both for the sake of clarity and also to aid curriculum planning. Skilbeck (1984) advocates using, as guides for learning, broad, comprehensive objectives which should not be confused with 'detailed inventories of pieces of behaviour'. Interestingly, the introduction to the Schools Council History 13–16 Project was based on a process model and provided broad objectives in the teachers' guide. For example, it was hoped the pupils would 'appreciate the tentative nature of many conclusions drawn from evidence' (Schools Council, 1976). Kelly (1989), however, firmly rejects objectives in any form. He argues that the starting point in educational planning should be a concern with what is known about the nature of children and with child development. Education, for Kelly, *is* development and it should be seen as a continuous experience which has no ends outside itself. So he rejects objectives because he sees them as instrumental, relating to ends which are separate from the educational process. One solution to this problem could be to formulate 'process objectives', i.e. objectives specifying what developmental processes it is hoped students will achieve. These, too, are rejected by Blenkin and Kelly (1987) because for them developmental qualities are not end-states, extrinsic to educational processes and activities. Thus the development of autonomy is not something which will be achieved at a later date if appropriate learning activities are organised at the present time. The development of autonomy is rather a principle which should permeate the pupil's whole educational experience (Blenkin and Kelly, 1987).

At the heart of much of the debate about the use of objectives in education lies the question of what is meant by 'objectives'. Since this is an area of contention in nursing, as well as general education, the debate will be explored a little further, starting with an examination of Eisner's (1975) expressive objectives. These objectives identify the type of 'educational encounter' a student is to have and the behaviour of the student at the end of the learning experience is not specified. The focus is what is meaningful and interesting to the student and diversity, not homogeneity, of response from students is required. Thus pupils could '. . . interpret the meaning of Paradise Lost' (Eisner, 1975). (An example in nursing education could be to explore the issue of client empowerment for nurses and nursing.) Lawton (1983) suggests that the word 'objective' here may be confusing since Eisner is clearly not concerned with measurable products. Eisner (1985) has, in fact, now changed the terminology and refers to expressive activities which lead to expressive outcomes. Blenkin and Kelly (1987) suggest that expressive objectives are really a statement of procedures or principles, and Kelly (1989) argues that 'many people are very confused in their thinking about objectives, so that they call what they are doing framing objectives but then proceed to make these of such a general kind that they are not objectives in the instructional and behavioural sense of the term at all, but rather expressive objectives or principles . . .'

The situation with regard to objectives is indeed confused, and is ideologically quite highly charged. Individual nurse teachers will have different views about the place of objectives in nursing education, some seeing them as having a positive contribution to make, and some wishing to reject them. However, as the above discussion suggests, the word 'objective' can be used to denote statements which have nothing in common with *behavioural* objectives. It is therefore worthwhile ending this section by trying to pull together the threads of the foregoing analysis in the context of nursing education.

The first point is the very practical one that in nursing education there are competencies to be achieved and students have to be assessed in relation to these competencies. In some cases the learning outcomes must be specific and it is in this area that behavioural objectives have a place. This does not mean that education has to be seen as an unpleasant mechanistic process of moulding students, and indeed students may very well be involved in planning their own objectives. The main point is that if certain achievements are required it is only fair that students and teachers should be aware of those requirements. Objectives are one way of facilitating this communication, and broad general objectives are usually an adequate guide. Rowntree (1982) describes various types of objectives including 'content objectives'. These relate to the concepts and principles associated with subject areas; in nursing education the required knowledge-content related to the concept 'adaptation' could be stated as a content objective. Rowntree (1982) also discusses 'methodological objectives' which refer to the particular methods of investigation and so on, which are associated with the subject disciplines. Objectives relating to the assessment, planning, implementation and evaluation of nursing care could be seen as examples in nursing education. A third group of objectives are those referring to 'life skills', which include affective objectives (Rowntree, 1982). In this group are included objectives such as those formulated by Carl Rogers in the area of 'self-actualisation': 'He becomes more self-confident and self-directing' (Rogers, 1961; cited by Rowntree, 1982).

Rowntree (1982) draws attention to the frequent use of words such as 'adequate' and 'more' in these 'infinitely improvable' sets of objectives, but argues very firmly that they are 'far more suggestive of appropriate teaching strategies and learning experiences than are the high-minded platitudes and woolly generalizations that usually preside over curriculum planning'. In nursing education it could be argued that such objectives, if used, should be generated by the student in the context of peer and pastoral support. Objectives relating to increasing self-confidence in some aspect of nursing practice could well form part of a learning contract.

Rowntree (1982) queries how realistic it is to separate life-skill and methodological objectives, and states that writers use the term 'process objectives' to include both methodological and life-skill objectives. Most process objectives are infinitely improvable and Rowntree (1982) argues that insufficient attention is paid to these objectives; the emphasis is on content. He cites Miller (1962) whose evaluation of the teaching and learning in the University of Illinois medical school indicated that though 'critical thinking' was considered an important aim (though not spelt out as objectives), nevertheless the students were given little opportunity to question and discuss and 'be critical'. This issue is very relevant to nursing education, with an increasing emphasis on the need for students to develop such skills as analysis, critical thinking, problem-solving and communication (UKCC, 1988). Some nurse teachers may prefer the terminology 'principles of procedure' or 'expressive activities' for some open-ended parts of the curriculum, but it is important they really are open-ended! For, as a University of London Curriculum Review Unit argues in the context of *teacher* education:

'... it would be mistaken to distinguish process-based approaches from product-based ones solely in terms of the tutor's methods; the real distinction lies in the principal aim of the course. If the aim is that every prospective teacher should know certain things, be familiar with debates, issues and literature within a specific field, and have mastered certain specific skills and professional practices then the course will be primarily product-based (however progressive the tutor's methods may be). By contrast, the principal aim of a process-based approach is not the transmission or acquisition of 'knowledge' (the results of the thinking of others) but is the development by student teachers of strategies for learning and improving the practice of teaching.'

(Porter, 1983)

The definition of product is broader than that already discussed in the context of the behavioural objectives model but the distinction made above is extremely significant. The sort of 'products' referred to have an important place in the education of nurses, but they are insufficient in themselves to equip practitioners for future practice in time of rapid change.

This discussion about different interpretations and approaches with regard to using objectives is by no means comprehensive, no mention having been made, for example, of Steinaker and Bell's (1979) experiential taxonomy. For interested readers, Kenworthy and Nicklin (1989) suggest how this taxonomy can assist in the planning of a nursing curriculum. However, an attempt has been made to discuss, in relation to different approaches to curriculum planning, some of the ways teaching intentions and learning outcomes can be expressed. The confusion seems most evident in relation to the process models, but turning from these, two cultural analysis models of curriculum planning will now be considered.

Planning by cultural analysis

Key exponents of this approach in general education are Lawton (1981; 1983) and Skilbeck (1975; 1984). Both are reconstructionists. Thus, Lawton (1983) embraces a 'democratic, non-Utopian version of social reconstructionism', believing that education can not only benefit individuals but can also be used to improve an imperfect society. He advocates a common curriculum and argues that in simple terms cultural analysis requires curriculum planners to ask the following questions:

'(a) What kind of society already exists?
 (b) In what ways is it developing?
 (c) How do its members appear to want it to develop?
 (d) What kinds of values and principles will be involved in deciding on (c) and on the educational means for achieving (c)?'

(Lawton, 1983)

By 'culture' Lawton (1983) means 'everything that is man-made in society: tools and technology, language and literature, music and art, science and mathematics, attitudes and values – in effect, the whole way of life of that society.' The task of curriculum planners is therefore to analyse and select from the culture the knowledge and experience most appropriate to meet the needs of individual pupils. Chapter 3 of this book provides a worked example of how an adapted version of Lawton's (1983) model can be used in conjunction with a nursing model to plan a paediatric nursing curriculum, while Gilling (1989) suggests how Lawton's model could be used to plan a common core curriculum for nurses, midwives and health visitors.

Skilbeck (1975) also advocates a common curriculum and a focus on the 'Study and appraisal of contemporary culture'. Such an approach requires emphasis on subjects such as sociology, politics, economics and environmental science, and teachers need experience in 'problem-solving, critical enquiry and creative activity' (Skilbeck, 1975). As Lawton (1983) points out, knowledge is not ignored in a reconstructionist curriculum, 'but a 'why' question is never far away'. Skilbeck (1982b) outlines an approach to curriculum planning, key elements of which are external and internal situational analyses. The external analysis focuses on factors external to the school which need to be considered in planning, and these include not only cultural and social changes but also factors such as the requirements of the educational system and resources available. The internal situational analysis is related to the school itself and focuses on aspects such as the perceived problems in the existing curriculum, the needs of pupils and the experience of teachers, the resources available and the ethos and political structure of the institution. The model also involves goal formulation, programme building, identification of possible problems in implementing curriculum change, as well as the design of assessment and evaluation schemes. Skilbeck (1984) states that these stages can be developed concurrently or even in reverse; the model does not imply that curriculum planners should follow a rigid step-by-step approach.

Skilbeck's (1982b; 1984) situational analysis model can easily be adapted for use in nursing education, and as Taylor and Richards (1985) suggest, it provides a framework 'which can encompass either the process model or the objective model depending on which aspects of the curriculum are being designed. It is flexible, adaptable and open to interpretation in the light of changing circumstances'. Chapter 2 of this book indicates how a situational analysis can assist in planning the ethics component of a Common Foundation Programme for Project 2000.

In the foregoing sections of this chapter the distinctive features of four ideologies have been discussed and the fourfold approach has been used to analyse several curriculum planning models. The next section draws on the previous discussion to suggest how the fourfold approach can help in the formulation of an educational philosophy in nursing education.

Formulating an educational philosophy

ENB (1989b) describe how a Director of Midwifery Education set about the task of creating a corporate identity for a new College of Midwifery which was formed by the amalgamation of five smaller schools. Workshops were held, and during the first of these an attempt was made to formulate an outline educational philosophy for the College. Before the workshop the 20 participants were asked to read some descriptions of educational philosophy which had been extracted from submission documents. Having reflected on what, as individuals, they wanted to see included in the College philosophy, they were to write down, briefly, on separate cards, the three most important things. During the workshop session the Gibson technique was used to 'explore consensus' about the College's educational philosophy. The prepared cards from each participant were placed face up on tables and the group circulated, turning over any they disagreed with. At the end the cards face up did not require discussion, because everyone agreed with the statements. Those which were face down needed to be discussed so that disagreement about the statements themselves or the wording could be explored. ENB (1989b) suggest that the technique involves everyone and saves wasting time in discussing areas of agreement. Cards *can* be prepared beforehand by one or two people, leaving a few blank ones for any additions by group members. However, ENB (1989b) argue that though this provides 'succinct relevant statements' people would be less involved.

It is interesting that, for some participants, thinking in philosophical terms was difficult and they would have liked *prepared* statements. Such statements would seem to have a further advantage, namely that they could be selected so as to represent a wide spectrum of beliefs. This is where a fourfold approach has something to offer. There is always the danger that, in summarising any ideology, distortion creeps in, but the following statements would seem to be reasonably representative of the four ideologies already discussed. The statements would not be classified in any way for a workshop activity and would be 'muddled up' on the tables, but here they are categorised using the following coding system: NE = role of nursing education; KJ = view of knowledge and justification for learning; T = role of teacher; C = content of curriculum; S = implicit view of student; CU = definition of curriculum. The four definitions of curriculum correspond to Skilbeck's (1984) 'design briefs' which underpin Beattie's (1987) Fourfold Curriculum, and which it has been suggested in this chapter correspond to the four ideologies discussed. The definitions interestingly illustrate how different ideologies result in quite different conceptions of what a curriculum actually *is*, but for the Gibson technique one or two might need rewording to make them more 'user friendly'!

The following provides 24 statements which could be used as a starting point for formulating an educational philosophy at an institutional level.

Instrumentalism

NE Nursing education should adapt to meet the changing needs of society.

KJ There is a right and a wrong way of performing a nursing skill and mastery of correct techniques is essential for safe practice and the protection of the public.

T Nurse teachers have a key role in training students in social and psychomotor skills.

C The acquisition of practical skills is vitally important.

S Students need demonstrations and plenty of supervised practice to master nursing skills.

CU The curriculum is 'a kind of technology – a pattern or design comprising clearly specified tasks for the teachers and students' (Skilbeck, 1984).

Liberal humanism

NE Nursing education should ensure that the body of worthwhile nursing knowledge is preserved and transmitted to the next generation.

KJ Some knowledge is relatively objective and timeless and should be acquired because the content is worthwhile in itself, not as a means to an end.

T Nurse teachers have expert knowledge which needs to be transmitted to students.

C Sound academic knowledge is fundamental to the nursing curriculum.

S Students need sound explanations to enable them to grasp fundamental knowledge concepts and principles.

CU The curriculum is 'a body or corpus of knowledge to be organized, communicated, acted upon and in some sense reproduced by students' (Skilbeck, 1984).

Progressivism

NE Nursing education should help students grow and develop.

KJ Knowledge is tentative and hypothetical and its worthwhileness depends on an individual student's response to it.

T Nurse teachers should facilitate meaningful personal experiences for students.

C Students should be free to study the things that interest them most.

S Students should be encouraged to be active and self-directed in their learning.

CU The curriculum 'is to be thought of in terms of activity and experience rather than of knowledge to be acquired and facts to be stored' (Hadow Report, 1931; cited by Skilbeck, 1984).

Reconstructionism

NE Nursing education should be a positive force in the creation of a better society.

KJ Knowledge involves exploring, for the good of society, problems and dilemmas which afflict society and to which solutions cannot be readily agreed.

T Nurse teachers have a responsibility to help students explore controversial cultural and political issues.

C An examination of current societal problems should form a key element in the nursing curriculum.

S Students should be encouraged to be critical and questioning in the way they view society.

CU The curriculum is a 'process of mapping – the means whereby students and teachers jointly structure, and restructure selected aspects of the culture' (Skilbeck, 1984).

In using the above statements for a workshop, blank cards could also be provided for extra statements by participants. If the meaning of any statement is unclear participants should turn the cards face down. It is useful at some point in the discussions about a philosophy to ensure that participants clarify, in concrete terms, the implications of their choice of statements. For example, the statement that students 'should be encouraged to be active and self-directed in their learning' can become so well-worn and the 'done thing' to accept, that the implications of such acceptance may not be fully explored! Yet when statements such as this have been agreed upon, they should be clearly reflected throughout the institution's curricula, otherwise the formulation of a philosophy becomes meaningless. The problem of different interpretations is well exemplified by the remarks of a Director of Nurse Education in relation to achieving a common philosophy and practice between two Schools of Nursing and Midwifery and a polytechnic: 'You can talk with each other for a considerable amount of time, thinking you're on the same lines, and the same phrases mean the same thing to both sides. And suddenly someone make a comment, and you realise that you were nowhere near each other' (cited by ENB, 1989b).

It is useful, too, to explore rejected statements carefully. Statement KJ for liberal humanism, for example, could very well end up face down! However, discussion about it could lead to the generation of ideas as to how necessary knowledge-content could be taught in satisfying ways which furthered students' personal as well as their professional development. It could also open up the way for the inclusion of liberal studies in the curriculum. In this way rejected statements could be modified into an acceptable form. In order to give participants time to reflect upon the statements it could be helpful to circulate the list beforehand and incorporate a rating scale so that participants were required to indicate whether they strongly agreed, agreed, disagreed or strongly disagreed with each statement. These papers would not be collected in at the workshop and this should be made clear to participants.

The discussion above has focused on how a fourfold approach can assist in formulating a strictly *educational* philosophy, but the Gibson card technique could be used to explore beliefs about such concepts as nursing, health, and the individual. Philosophical statements relating, for example, to a Common Foundation Programme and branch programmes should be congruent with the institutional philosophy, but would be more specific. An example of a philosophy related to care of the child is given in Chapter 3.

In the next section of this chapter the fourfold theme will be continued at a much more concrete level. Suggestions will be made as to how content and learning experiences can be selected and organised, and the implications for the design of assessment schemes will be explored. The discussion will focus on the development of a Project 2000 Common Foundation Programme (CFP), but reference will also be made to branch programmes.

Developing a four dimensional curriculum model

In analysing UKCC's (1986; 1988) outlines of future pre-registration preparation, a number of themes emerge. First, there is an emphasis on a sound *knowledge* base, which includes the biological, physical and social sciences and the humanities, and is applied to nursing theory and practical *experience*. The body of knowledge for the CFP must be 'embedded in health as well as in illness' and must be part of a practice based curriculum (UKCC, 1988). Second, in relation to the CFP, reference is made to what could be called *general 'developmental processes'* such as analytical skills, critical thinking, communication skills, problem-solving and working in teams. For branch programmes further processes are identified, for example coping with emotions and 'observing, interpreting and reporting behaviour, feelings and attitudes' (UKCC, 1988). More specific CFP skills are also identified, such as handling patients and equipment. Third, for both CFP and branch programmes, students must have experience in a *range of settings* with, fourth, a *variety of clients and patients* and with individuals, families, groups and communities.

So four key dimensions of future pre-registration preparation are the provision of practical experience underpinned by a sound knowledge base, taking place in a range of settings with a variety of clients and patients, and with the whole programme being permeated by an emphasis on general developmental processes. The four dimensions are closely inter-related but it could be helpful from a planning point of view to separate them in order to highlight their importance. The term 'general developmental processes' has been chosen to indicate those processes which are not particularly associated with any specific part of the curriculum. For example, processes such as lifting and handling patients are specific to practice settings, whereas critical thinking, though important in such settings, has a much more general application.

The dimensions discussed above are similar to those described for a core curriculum for Australian schools (Curriculum Development Centre (CDC), 1982; Skilbeck, 1984; 1985). Skilbeck (1985) describes three dimensions: 'areas of knowledge and experience', 'learning environments' and 'learning processes'. According to CDC (1982) the first area includes a range of core learnings which embody theoretical content and practical experiences. For example, health education includes the study of human biology and nutrition and also programmes of sport and relaxation. The second area, learning environments, emphasises the need to provide a variety of settings, for example classrooms, small group learning spaces and fieldwork (Skilbeck, 1985). The third dimension, learning processes, includes 'learning and thinking techniques such as problem-solving, lateral thinking, organised study habits', 'ways of organising knowledge such as ... gathering and interpreting evidence' and 'interpersonal and group relationships' (CDC, 1982). These learning processes are ones which are available through different experiences and subjects.

Continuing with this approach, it would seem that Beattie's (1987) Fourfold Curriculum, underpinned by the four ideologies, encompasses the 'areas of knowledge and experience'. Intimately related to this dimension are two others, namely, 'a range of settings and a variety of clients and patients'. A fourth dimension is that of 'developmental processes' which has been chosen in preference to 'learning processes' because the latter can become confused with learning *activities* such as reading or writing (which may not necessarily involve any development!). Putting these elements together, in effect, results in a Four

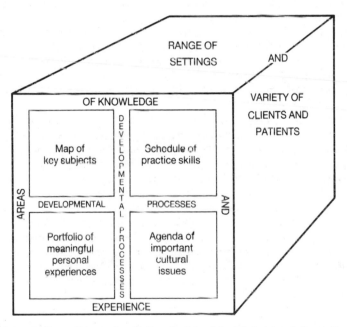

Fig. 1.1 A Four Dimensional Curriculum Model (adapted from Beattie's (1987) Fourfold Curriculum and Curriculum Development Centre's (1982) Three Dimensional Core Curriculum).

Dimensional Curriculum Model (Fig. 1.1). The model bears a curious resemblance to a Battenberg cake and provided this analogy is not pressed too far, it serves as a reminder that teaching, learning and curriculum planning should be so enjoyable that people come back for more!

Some worked examples as to how the model could be used will be discussed but, before doing so, the four dimensions require some further exploration.

Areas of knowledge and experience

It is suggested that the 'areas of knowledge and experience' encompass Beattie's (1987) Fourfold Curriculum and its underlying ideologies. Beattie (1987) discusses the four approaches and their advantages and limitations and there is no intention here to repeat his arguments. A few brief points, though, will be made. Beattie (1987) refers to one approach as drawing up 'a schedule of basic skills', which he defines as 'those areas of practical competence which are deemed to be essential for responsible and effective performance of professional tasks'. He suggests that the nursing process can form a framework for the teaching of such basic skills. However, in the light of earlier discussion in this chapter about instrumentalism and the training of health care assistants (see p.4), it could be argued that the term 'basic skills' is problematic. 'Basic skills' in the future could refer to those skills required by health care assistants.

The NCVQ framework will require curriculum planners to think in terms of different *levels* of skilled performance, and for this reason 'practice skills' has been included in Fig. 1.1. Beattie (1987) also discusses subject-mapping as an approach to curriculum planning and it has been suggested in this chapter that this is associated with liberal humanism. Interestingly, Beattie suggests that drawing up a schedule of basic skills and subject-mapping both embody a definition of knowledge as 'authoritative', 'consensual' and 'closed'. He also considers curriculum as a 'portfolio of meaningful personal experiences', an approach which involves organising and sequencing the curriculum around the students' interests and on 'the practical and concrete situations (in their personal and professional lives) that they find most puzzling or troubling'. Beattie (1987) provides several examples of how opportunities for students to discuss their experiences can be built into the curriculum. Such an approach is associated with a progressivist ideology. Finally, Beattie (1987) explores the fourth approach which emphasises 'dilemmas and debates' on an agenda of open-ended cultural issues, and which offers a problem-solving means of keeping up to date with current affairs. It is suggested here that this approach is related to a reconstructionist ideology. Beattie (1987) stresses the 'conditional' and 'open' definition of knowledge inherent in the last two approaches.

All four elements of the Fourfold Curriculum embody various 'developmental processes', many of which are of a general nature. It is to highlight their importance that they are considered here as a distinct, but inter-related, dimension. The following section suggests how some general developmental processes can be fostered.

Developmental processes

Squires (1987) suggests that making a distinction between content and process is helpful in clarifying the concepts of 'level' and 'difficulty'. To some extent higher and more difficult levels of work and study require a student to 'know more', in terms of more knowledge of the subject literature and the acquisition of more advanced skills. But, he argues, 'level and difficulty are also and more critically a matter of process; of how one engages with content'. It would, for example, be possible for a student to handle complex issues in a purely descriptive way. Squires' (1987) comments are particularly relevant for curriculum planners in nursing education at a time when academic accreditation is being sought for nursing qualifications.

Not surprisingly, Kelly (1989) advocates careful planning in order to facilitate developmental processes. He gives an example related to the development of literary awareness and suggests that teachers should identify clearly what literary awareness means and what its key elements and processes are. Principles of procedure can then be formulated and appropriate work and activities planned. With regard to the development of critical thinking in nurses Brookfield (1987) has much to offer. He includes material on what critical thinking means, how to recognise it, what its components are and how to facilitate its development. A chapter on media literacy suggests how television interviews, newspapers and so on can be analysed for bias and distortion.

The focus in this discussion, however, is on using writing as a means of facilitating developmental processes. Allen *et al.* (1989) draw the distinction between 'writing as recording thought' and 'writing as developing thinking'. In the former, the skills of thinking and writing are seen as different, and knowing something precedes writing about it. By contrast, the notion of 'writing as developing thinking' or 'writing to learn' assumes that writing is a process by which understanding can be developed. Writing is seen as involving an inner dialogue and each new draft furthers the student's understanding of the content. Allen *et al.* (1989) argue that literacy

'in the fullest sense is the creating and organizing of thoughts, the sorting of assertions and relevant evidence, and the development of and support for reasoned decision making. If our graduate nurses are going to be able to respond to the rapidly changing health-care system, deliver professional care and justify its importance when competing for limited funds, they must have these cognitive skills.'

(Allen *et al.*, 1989)

One approach to 'writing to learn' is to encourage students to keep journals (Allen *et al.*, 1989). Holly and McLoughlin (1989) discuss journal writing in the context of teacher professional development but what they say has equal relevance for nurses. Journals include facts, possibly feelings and thoughts, and they involve a systematic and comprehensive attempt at clarification of ideas and experience. They help practitioners to look back and reflect on their experiences, and can assist in coming to grips with problems (Holly and McLoughlin, 1989). Hahnemann (1986) used journals to encourage students to write on set topics, for example 'Take one sentence from your readings that sparked your interest and write on its meaning'. She also used the journals to facilitate the expression of feelings, in order to help the students cope better with stresses and frustrations. Such exercises could be very helpful in furthering the students' emotional development. This use of journals is associated with what Holly (1988; cited by Holly and McLoughlin, 1989) calls 'therapeutic writing', an approach which includes catharsis, humour and self-analysis. Journals can be purely private affairs, or they can be used in discussion with peers and teachers. They can also be used as an assessment tool and reference will be made to this later in the chapter.

A different approach to written assignments is adopted by Sobralske (1989). She asks student nurses to choose a health promotion topic related to any client age group and write a three page paper suitable for reading by the general public. Topics chosen included 'care of contact lenses', 'dealing with adolescent stress' and 'preventing skin cancer'. Articles have been published in local newspapers, the university student newspaper, and a hospital newsletter. On a similar theme, students were given health related questions from advice columns and were asked to write suitable responses (Cooper, 1986).

An ingenious approach to facilitating learning about drug actions which involves creative writing and speaking, is described by Lantz and Meyers (1986) and involves the use of personification. Included below are the instructions given to students and an example of one student's work:

'Since drugs exhibit many unique characteristics, one can almost view them as people. They belong to a family and assume characteristics of the family, but still are unique. From the following given list, select one drug and describe it as if it were you. Include the following:
1. family and family characteristics;
2. your unique characteristics;
3. what you do and whom do you work with best;
4. interaction problems;
5. adverse reactions.'

Lantz and Meyers (1986) then describe the student.

'... entering the classroom in a long white robe and a turban on his head sitting on the desk with crossed legs. As he begins to intone what he has written, he becomes Valium:
'Ooommmm! My name is Val. I come from India. I am your Guru. Take me, I'll show you the way – I'll show you peace, love, inner harmony and tranquillity. The truth of my ways can be seen by my popularity – I give peace and am most loved of drugs – I am the #1 of all prescribed drugs in the U.S. of A. I am known to many as Diazepam, of the house of Benzodiazepines, and am the eldest and most loved of my family – the antianxiety drugs – perhaps you know my brothers, Librium, Xanax. All of us reach your soul, affect your mind, brothers and sisters, for we are psychotropic drugs. Are you tense, anxious, tired, or agitated? Let me show you the light, the promise of holy peace, the glimpse of Nirvana. If life is too tough, come to me, come into my embrace of tranquillity. I'll relax your large skeletal muscles and have a direct effect on your brain and effect the essence of being, brother. I will be your chief Guru, listen to my lessons and avoid the Gurus of alcohol, narcotics, barbiturates, MAO inhibitors, antihistamines, sleeping pills, tranquillizers for our paths to inner peace may conflict I am the light, the peace, the calm, my lessons can be heavysome, especially the old and weak may become sleepy and drowsy in my light. Don't drive or operate machinery when you are on the enlightened plane with me. For some, the message of inner peace is too great and they become confused, depressed, disoriented, have headaches, changes in sex drive, slurred speech. None of my pupils may have narrow angle glaucoma, for my light will blind the unprepared. I come in white, yellow and blue tablets or take me directly into your veins or flesh – 40 mg a day for an adult is my maximum strength. Take me – have inner peace. For this reason I am over loved by some. Many of my pupils abuse my gifts, others who try to live without me suffer withdrawal symptoms such as sweating, convulsions, tremors, muscle cramps and vomiting. I am loved, I am peace, I am inner tranquillity – escape the woes of your hectic world. I am the way to inner calm. I am your Guru. I am Val. Ooommmm!'

Dave Dickens, RN, BSN
(From Lantz and Meyers, 1986)

The above examples suggest how some general developmental processes can be fostered through writing. Such activities give students an opportunity to exercise imagination and creativity and as Brookfield (1987) points out, by 'recognising how their powers of imagination have been engaged, people begin to realise that they possess creative, speculative capacities and that they can call on these for a variety of purposes'. There is certainly a need in curriculum planning to identify key developmental processes and ensure that they are built into the curriculum. Journals seem to be a particularly effective approach since they can be used for analysis, evaluation, reflection, introspection, and as a therapeutic tool (Holly, 1988; cited by Holly and McLoughlin, 1989). Furthermore journals can help link theory and practice, and could be a means of providing continuity between the CFP and branch programmes. However, future pre-registration students will also be required to have experience in a range of settings and with a variety of clients and patients.

Learning in a range of settings and with a variety of clients and patients

UKCC (1986) suggested that placements for students undertaking Common Foundation and branch programmes should be based on different age groups or client/patient needs, or on concepts such as pain or stress. A variety of settings was to be selected and could include such areas as hospital wards, residential homes, slimming clubs and the workplace. Oliver (1988) describes a new course curriculum developed for mental handicap nursing in the context of a community-based service. With the shift away from hospital provision the traditional placements of students with different categories of people (children, adults, and so on) were no longer possible. Instead, the placements are based on themes such as 'normalisation, individual programme planning, communication skills and working with families' (Oliver, 1988). To overcome the problem of travelling to far distant placements, students are attached to specially created bases in urban centres nearest their homes.

Allor (1983) describes a community profile tool for students to use during their community placements. The tool includes characteristics of the population (ethnic groups, sex and age distributions and so on); population facilities (for example, availability of playgrounds and shops); the environment (air, transport, sanitation, housing and industry); and a health profile (including health care facilities, what the public see as health problems, health statistics). Students are required to judge the effect, for good or ill, of each factor on the health of the community. Allor (1983) considers that the community profile helps develop observation skills and that the whole exercise 'fosters curiosity, healthy independence and resourcefulness, and creative investigation'.

Dobson (1986) advocates mini-ethnographic studies as a way of developing cultural awareness and sensitivity. Such studies require students to exercise skills of observation, participation and interviewing in a cultural setting, and help them become familiar with qualitative research methods. Dobson (1986) suggests that a group of students can work at one project, focusing for example on child-rearing practices.

An innovative scheme for taking health information to the public is described by Martin (1989), and could provide very good experience for students undertaking relevant branch programmes, if adequate support could be mustered. Martin (1989) explains how a group of health visitors have set up a thriving stall at the local market, at which consultations and free health literature are available. Involvement in a project such as this would provide students with valuable experience in patient teaching in a very informal setting. Links with schools would provide experience of the school health service and could perhaps open the way for students to give group presentations on health related topics. Student presentations could also be offered to local mother and baby clubs, young wives groups, scouts and guides, over 60s clubs and so on.

The provision of adequate support and broad experience for students in the community is discussed by Orr (1988) who suggests the setting up of community nursing centres which could link schools of nursing, institutions of higher and further education and community services. Such centres would focus on practice and research and would develop innovative approaches to health promotion in the community. She suggests students could run health programmes in day centres or provide a drop-in service for well elderly people. These activities could begin during the Common Foundation Programme and continue in branch programmes.

The scheme described by Howden and Baggaley (1989) could also provide very valuable community experience. Each student is allocated to a well elderly person whom she or he visits eight times during a six month period. Her or his role is not to provide health care or advice but to be 'an interested, caring observer'. The students also carry out four interviews with those involved with elderly people either professionally or in a voluntary capacity. This helps to broaden the students' understanding of the problems and needs of elderly people. A written health assessment of the elderly person is submitted as an assignment at the end of six months (Howden and Baggaley, 1989).

The discussion so far has centred on providing a variety of experiences for students in their community placements. However, Archer (1988) describes how students allocated to an acute psychiatric unit for their occupational therapy experience in effect took their clients into the community. Outings into the community are not new but what was different about this scheme was that students were supernumerary and their allocation was self-directed. They liaised with occupational therapists rather than being supervised by them, and their supernumerary status and freedom to work flexible hours meant they could offer clients social and therapeutic activities 'on an unprecedented scale', and in a range of settings. The experience helped them develop their organising abilities, and group and communication skills.

The preceding section has expanded on the curricular dimensions 'areas of knowledge and experience', 'developmental processes' and 'range of settings and a variety of clients and patients'. In the next part of this chapter some worked examples will be discussed to suggest how the Four Dimensional Model could assist in curriculum planning.

Planning for Project 2000

The ENB (1989c) guidelines for developing future pre-registration courses specify that the Common Foundation Programme must be 'embedded in the study of health focusing on nursing and emphasising its dynamic nature'. There is an emphasis on the acquisition of 'knowledge of a range of core subjects and skills', general development processes such as 'intellectual abilities, self-awareness and self-direction', and experience in a range of settings and with a variety of clients and patients. The following five basic concepts are to form the major themes of the Common Foundation Programme: the individual, society, health, health care and nursing. ENB (1989c) suggest possible content for each of these concepts.

These guidelines bring into sharper focus the general recommendations laid down by the UKCC's (1986) key document *Project 2000. A New Preparation for Practice*. A substantial part of this document represents, in effect, the results of a very large scale situational analysis at a macro level. Factors external to nursing and nursing education are considered, such as social change and its effect on health needs, and specific demographic change affecting recruitment to nursing. Internal factors relate to deficiencies in the current preparation of nursing and the problems of manpower wastage.

These factors are still relevant but the broad context of nursing education continues to change and exert an influence on curriculum planning in individual schools/colleges of nursing education, so that an external and internal situational analysis is also a crucial aspect of curriculum planning at local level. Indeed, such planning always has to be seen in the context of international, national and local trends, issues and forces. At an international level the World Health Organisation's target date for 'Health for All' is getting ever closer. However, as McFarlane (1989) points out, the Government's White Paper on the National Health Service, 'Working for Patients', puts little emphasis on health promotion and disease prevention. This is in spite of the conclusions of Whitehead's (1988) report 'The Health Divide', which suggests that 'serious social inequalities in health have persisted into the 1980s' in Britain. The report notes, however, the many efforts being made by health authorities and health workers to counteract such inequalities. The teaching of health promotion skills, then, constitutes a real challenge for nurse educators as we move into the 1990s, and in view of the current climate, there is an increasing need for students to develop political alertness.

The year 1992, also, is likely to have an influence on nursing curricula in the United Kingdom. Lyall (1989) predicts that following the creation of a single European market there is likely to be an increased flow of workers to and from the Continent, and that cultural differences in health care provision may well become increasingly interesting to nurses. During the 1990s, the problems of recruitment and retention of staff will remain a key concern, and shortages of qualified practitioners may pose a real threat to the provision of adequate support and supervision for students in practice settings. Pearce (1988) discusses various ways of trying to address these problems, including open days in schools/ colleges of nursing, designing more flexible programmes to meet the needs of mature students with family commitments and making contacts with career teachers in schools. It is to be hoped that the reform of nursing education will do much to make nursing more attractive to prospective entrants, and will reduce student wastage.

The above discussion has outlined only a few of the general contextual issues which influence the curriculum planning process. At local level the major tasks of amalgamating schools, forming links with institutions of higher education and seeking joint academic and professional validation for courses makes the curriculum planning process complex and exacting. Some aspects of educational change will be discussed at the end of this chapter, but the intention now is to consider how curriculum planners might set about the task of developing a Common Foundation Programme from the five key concepts specified by ENB (1989c): the individual, society, health, health care and nursing.'

Elaborating the key concepts

One way of elaborating the five concepts is to draw a concept map. Initially it is better not to study the ENB (1989c) suggestions for possible content but rather to give free rein to ideas that happen to flow. The aim is to maximise intellectual freedom and opportunities for creativity. Rowntree (1985) suggests that concept maps can help highlight possible connections between ideas. He advocates writing the ideas down on a large sheet of paper or whiteboard, or else jotting them on cards and moving them around on a table. After generating ideas and sorting out possible relationships, the ENB's (1989c) suggested content can be consulted to see if any broad areas which should be included are missing from the concept map. Figs 1.2–1.6 show the five concepts elaborated in a 'raw form'. They are only intended as examples and need much more refinement and further elaboration in the light of an institution's own situational analysis. Moreover, they are the effort of only one person (the author); in a planning operation a team of people should be involved, and they could formulate quite different maps from those illustrated. Having mapped out the five concepts, it could then be helpful to look for areas where ideas interrelate *between* concept areas and these could be marked with a highligher pen. It should now be possible to start organising a possible structure for the course.

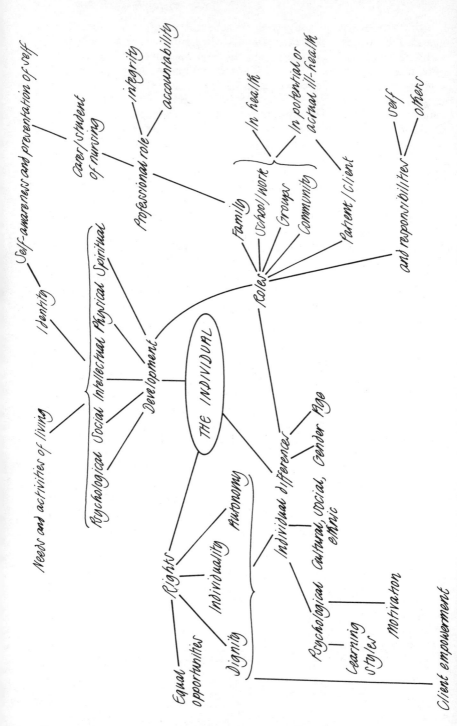

Fig. 1.2 Map to elaborate key concept 'the individual'

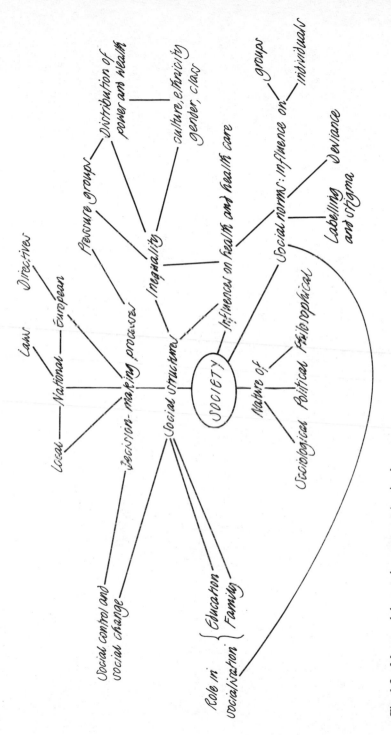

Fig. 1.3 Map to elaborate key concept 'society'.

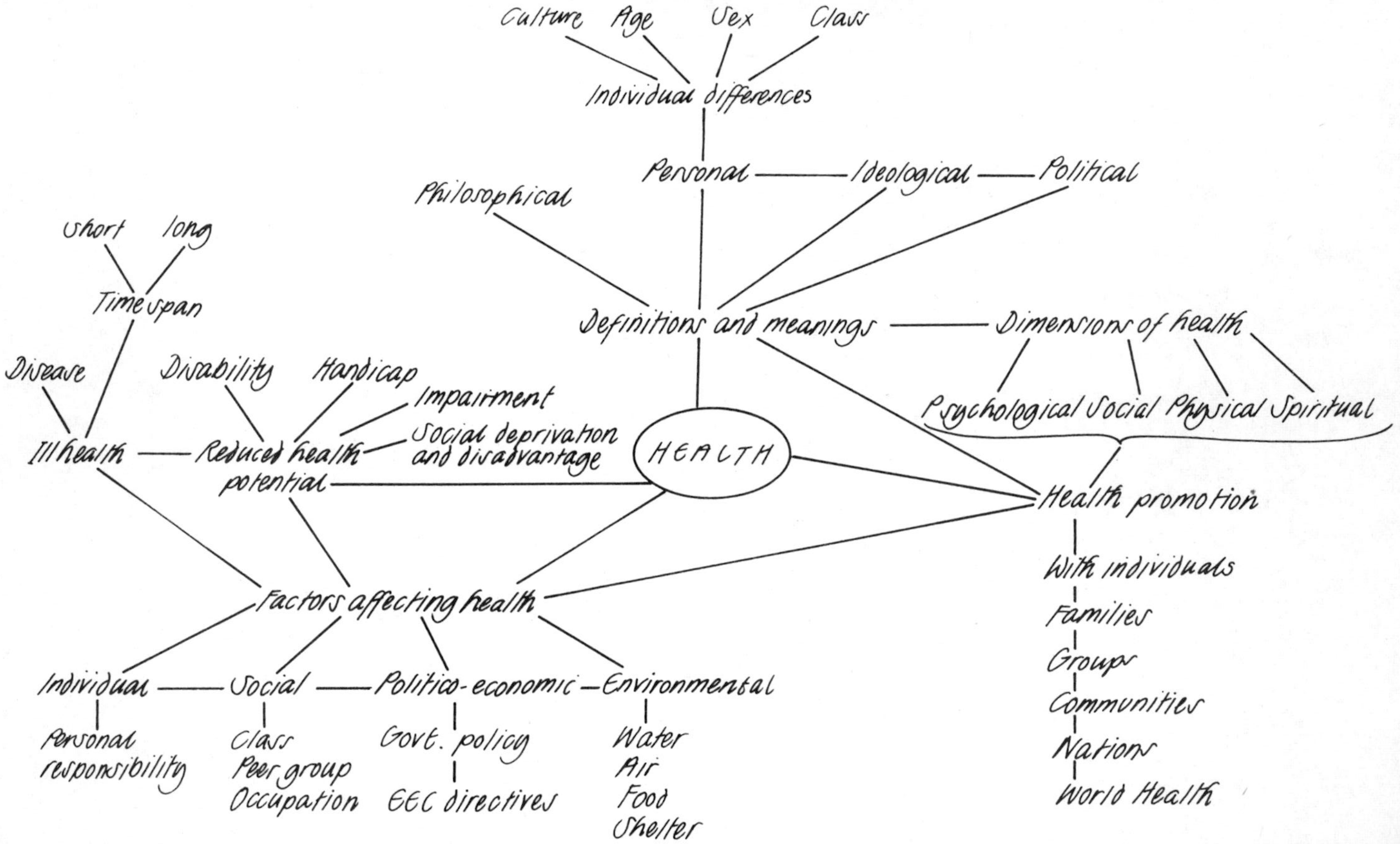

Fig. 1.4 Map to elaborate key concept 'health'.

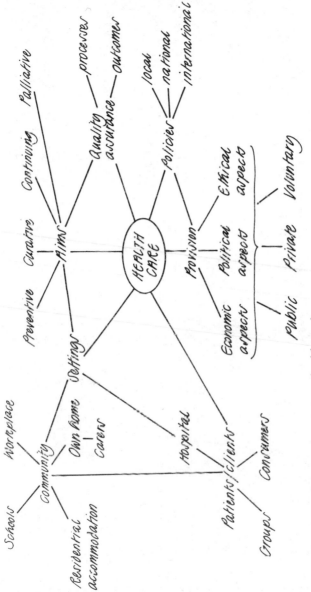

Fig. 1.5 Map to elaborate key concept 'health care'.

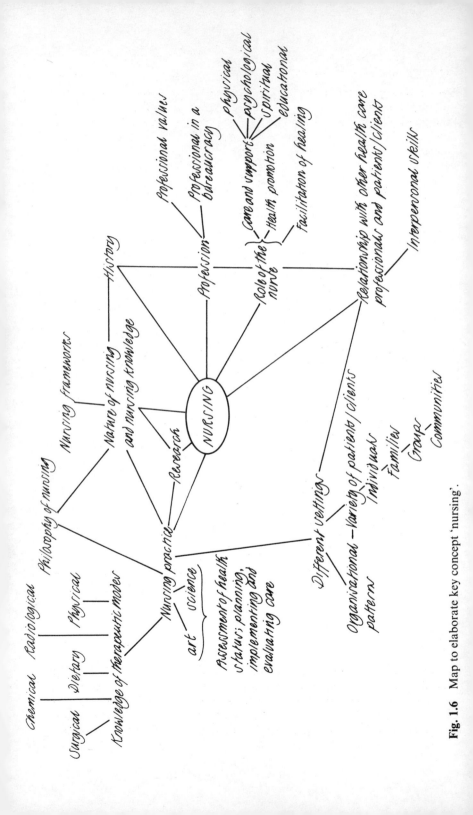

Fig. 1.6 Map to elaborate key concept 'nursing'.

Developing a course structure

When the concept maps have taken shape it may be possible to identify major themes which encompass all the ideas on each map. For example, the main all-encompassing themes in Figs 1.2, 1.3, 1.4 and 1.5 respectively, could be: individual differences, societal influences, health needs and health care provision. These could become vertical threads running through the Common Foundation Programme with nursing theory and

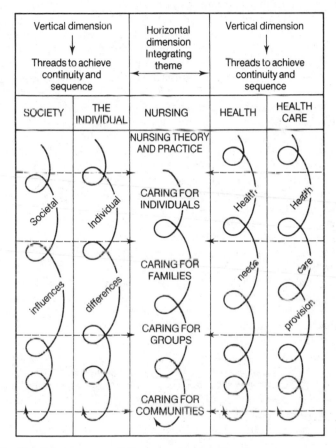

Fig. 1.7 Possible structure of Common Foundation Programme.

practice forming a central integrating core (Fig. 1.7). ENB (1989c) specify that the Common Foundation Programme must focus on nursing and emphasise its dynamic nature. The 'caring' element is also stressed in the guidelines and UKCC (1988) state that care should relate to individuals, families, groups and communities. In Fig. 1.7 nursing theory, practice and 'caring' are of central importance and continue throughout the course and at an increasing depth and breadth. Thus in Tyler's (1949) terms, continuity and sequence are facilitated, that is, the major nursing elements are not only reiterated throughout the course (continuity) but are explored in increasing depth and breadth (sequence). The organising principle here is related to the range of caring, from the specific to the general, i.e. from the individual to communities. Caring could be explored in a number of ways, for example in relation to nursing models. Thus, caring could be linked with the promotion of independence in individual patients or clients and could lead eventually to consideration of how independence could be promoted for groups in the community. Promoting independence at this level, for example, could involve nurses working with community groups to try and procure transport facilities for housebound elderly people.

In organising learning situations where students are involved in caring for individuals, families and communities, Allen (1977) advocates analysing the *complexity* of such situations according to a number of dimensions. An adapted version of Allen's analysis is shown in table form in Fig. 1.8. Thus assessing, planning, implementing and evaluating care for the individual is clearly less complex than doing the same for a community. Allen (1977) suggests that students may be involved in complex situations early in their course in order to broaden their experience and indeed one would want to facilitate the development of interpersonal skills throughout a course. Allen's (1977) analysis, however, helps to pinpoint some areas likely to be demanding, and potentially more stressful, for students.

Returning to Fig. 1.7, caring could also focus on the nurse as a healer, educator, advocate and so on. The spiralling on the nursing core indicates flexibility. For example, it would be possible to go through the sequence 'individual to community' twice, once in relation to wellness and then with the focus on illness. Alternatively, the sequence could be from the well and ill individual to families, groups and communities in health and illness. The backward spiral also shows that when caring for groups the *individual* element is never lost. This is reinforced by the 'individual differences' thread running through the course as an insistent reminder of the uniqueness of all human beings: patients, clients, relatives and carers. In Fig. 1.7 the elements forming the vertical threads *could* be the four ENB (1989c) concepts, but it is suggested that expanding these bare concepts a little makes them more meaningful. So Fig. 1.7 shows one possible embryo structure for a Common Foundation Programme. The core nursing element runs through the whole course and also serves as a theme which integrates the other four elements. At some point in the planning process decisions about division of the course into units and terms have to be made. In the next section a worked example is given to show how the Four

DIMENSIONS OF COMPLEXITY	Lower complexity ←———— LEARNING SITUATIONS ————→ Higher complexity ————→
	INCREASING DEMAND ON STUDENT
Number of people	One patient/client ———————————————— A community
Visibility	Physical states ———————————— Social and psychological states
Stability	Wellness ————————————————— Acute illness
Skills	Psychomotor ———————————————— Interpersonal
Knowledge	Specific diseases —————————— General health promotion
Attitudes	Morally uncontentious ———————————— Morally contentious

Fig. 1.8 The complexity of learning situations (adapted from Allen, 1977).

Dimensional Model could be used to select content and learning experiences.

Selecting and organising content and learning experiences

Figure 1.9 illustrates in broad terms how the Four Dimensional Curriculum could be used to select and organise content and learning experiences for teaching 'playing' as an activity of living. Some of the areas could be introduced in the Common Foundation Programme and then the theme 'playing' could be continued into the Child Branch Programme. This sort of approach would help improve the cohesion between the CFP and branch programme. The matrix would need further elaboration but it suggests how the four concept threads shown in Fig. 1.7 (p.39) could 'feed into' the central core element of nursing. The content and learning experiences shown in Fig. 1.9 can in turn be traced back to elements of the concept maps (Figs. 1.2–1.6, pp.34–38). The Four Dimensional Model helps ensure that an educational philosophy (based on the four ideologies) permeates the course, and that there is an emphasis on general developmental processes and the facilitation of wide ranging experiences.

This discussion has focused on planning Common Foundation and branch programmes, but the four dimensional approach could be used for other courses. For example, in planning a short ENB course a matrix could be drawn up, with the course objectives down the left hand column and the areas of knowledge and experience, developmental processes and range of settings and clients across the top. The Four Dimensional Model is also relevant in the planning of assessment schemes, and this will be the focus of the next part of this chapter.

Assessment of students

In a way it is artificial to consider assessment of students separately from the earlier discussion about facilitating developmental processes and organising experiences in a range of settings and with a variety of clients and patients. For as Rowntree (1987) advises, where possible 'assess 'naturalistically', concentrating on processes and products pursued for their own educational sakes rather than devising exercises solely for assessment purposes and not themselves meant to be learning experiences'. Bearing this in mind, the following discussion will explore what a four dimensional approach can offer curriculum planners in designing schemes of assessment.

	AREAS OF KNOWLEDGE AND EXPERIENCE				GENERAL DEVELOPMENTAL PROCESSES	RANGE OF SETTINGS	VARIETY OF CLIENTS/PATIENTS
ACTIVITY OF LIVING	PRACTICE SKILLS	KEY SUBJECTS	MEANINGFUL PERSONAL EXPERIENCES	IMPORTANT CULTURAL ISSUES	PROCESSES	SETTINGS	CLIENTS/PATIENTS
PLAYING Individual child	Assessing well child's play needs at different ages, planning, implementing and evaluating play provision	Child psychology – play and development	Activities chosen by students, for example: interview children of different ages and sexes for child's view of what play means		Observing Organising Communicating Analysing	Home, well baby clinics, play group, school	Children of different ages, sexes, cultures, ethnic groups, who are well, ill, disabled, handicapped
Family	Teaching parent(s)/future parents these skills	Educational psychology; Sociology—cultural and ethnic differences	Design toys Critical incident analysis	Family poverty and its affect on play provision and child development	Creating Reporting Reflecting	Home, hospital, residential home	
Special groups (ill-health, handicap, disability)	Assessing needs, planning, implementing and evaluating play provision and teaching parent(s) and carers these skills	Knowledge of illness, handicap, disability			Critical thinking		Parents and carers – actual and potential
Community	Assessing current provision, identifying ways of improving and a possible action plan	Sociology – urban deprivation. Child psychology		Play deprivation and its effects on community	Evaluating	Whole community; playgrounds, youth clubs and so on	

Fig. 1.9 Matrix planning using the Four Dimensional Curriculum Model.

Assessing areas of knowledge and experience

In the area of practice skills a vital concern must always be to try and ensure competent performance, and indeed for the instrumentalist protection of the public would be a key purpose of assessment in nursing education. However, mammoth lists of behavioural objectives are unlikely to be helpful to students or teachers not least because 'as competencies are broken down into more and more discrete subskills we tend to lose sight of the overall picture, so that we run the risk of assessing students on their ability to perform discrete observable skills rather than to deliver effective care to the whole patient' (Ewan and White, 1984). Wysocki (1980) refers to the 'unique mix of head, heart and hands that is nursing practice' and notes that a 'variety of elements integrate to form the whole. Some of these are easily observed, documented and assessed and others are so subtle they may easily pass unseen'. It could be argued that behavioural objectives have a limited place in the assessment of practical skills but a key problem is the assumption that behaviour can be broken down and measured in a scientific and 'objective' way. According to this scientific paradigm, Guba and Lincoln (1981; cited by Simons, 1987) assert, reality is seen as 'singular, convergent and fragmentable'. One solution in nursing is the use of graded competency statements which at the highest level incorporate the competencies required of a qualified nurse. A worked example can be found in Skelton (1989).

With regard to the future pre-registration preparation of nurses, ENB (1989c) state that the Common Foundation and Branch Programme will normally be one continuous educational process and that assessment strategies must be continuing and must relate to theory and practice. The opportunities of integrating learning and assessment are certainly enhanced by these requirements. It is, however, essential that students clearly understand which elements of the course count towards their final result and are therefore primarily summative, and which elements are purely formative and designed to further their learning.

Turning from an instrumentalist ideology which stresses practical competence for the provision of a safe public service, we shall consider next the implications of assessment from a liberal humanist perspective. The emphasis in this ideology is on acquiring knowledge which is intrinsically worthwhile or which helps develop the intellect. Earlier in this chapter suggestions were made as to what liberal humanism could offer nursing education. Here just two points will be made. First, Hirst (1974) emphasises the importance of students understanding concepts, and Peters (1966) argues that one of the features of being 'educated' is having a body of knowledge and some understanding of 'principles for the organization of facts', and of the 'reason why' of things. Such knowledge should not be inert; it should transform a person's outlook on life around him. These ideals are pertinent to nursing education and point to the importance of assessing students' understanding and application of nursing related concepts such as 'independence' and the principles of asepsis and so on. Such concepts and principles underpin nursing practice and can be assessed by means of care studies or written questions as well as in practice settings.

The second point is related to the first and concerns one of Jarvis's (1983) criteria for the selection of curriculum content. He argues that one of the aims of professional education is the development of critical awareness of subjects taught and that this requires students to study these subjects in sufficient depth. 'Depth' here could refer to the sort of understanding of concepts and principles advocated by Hirst (1974) and Peters (1966). Indeed Peters (1966) suggests that vocational training (he would include professional preparation here) can also be *educational* if disciplines are taught in such a way that the student begins to grasp 'from the inside' what the particular form of thought entails. Jarvis's (1983) argument suggests that students should be required in the assessments to demonstrate a critical approach to subject matter.

The two ideologies discussed so far in relation to student assessment are both associated with somewhat teacher dominant approaches to assessment and relatively closed views of knowledge. Progressivism, however, places the student at the centre of learning and assessment processes and the emphasis would be on formative assessement. It could be argued that this is an aspect of progressivism with which Stenhouse (1975) would agree, for he argues in the context of a process model that in one sense 'assessment is about the teaching of self-assessment'. He argues this in relation to those areas of the curriculum which are concerned with knowledge and understanding, rather than information and skills. However, in nursing education self-assessment in all areas of the curriculum is to be encouraged, for as Heron (1988) stresses, self and peer assessment is 'the central way of maintaining and developing standards of professional practice'. Self-assessment can be facilitated by the use of journals and Burnard (1988) discusses various options for this. They can, for instance, be used purely formatively as an ongoing focus of discussion between student and teacher or ward manager. An example of this approach is given in Chapter 2. They can also be used as a summative assessment at the end of a clinical placement or in conjunction with peer evaluation.

The progressivist ideology with its emphasis on 'meaningful personal experiences' (Beattie, 1987) seems also to point to contract learning as a way of maximising choice for students in their assessments. As de Tornyay and Thompson (1987) suggest, this approach recognises the individuality of the student; the need for adults to be self-directing in their learning; the belief in students' accountability and responsibility for their learning; and the recognition of learning as a lifelong process. Chapter 7 of this book includes discussion of the use of learning contracts in nursing education. The reconstructionist ideology shares progressivism's open view of knowledge but is society orientated. Essays or seminars on topical cultural issues in nursing could be appropriate assessment strategies. Extracts from the Health Service Commissioner's (Ombudsman) reports could be analysed and students could be required to speculate on the underlying issues involved in the various scenarios and offer suggestions for improvements. They could also choose a letter from the professional or general press relating to a politico-ethical issue in nursing or health care and analyse and comment on the assumptions made and the arguments put forward. The important thing is to ensure that students have an opportunity to explore ideas in an open-ended way, and this in turn will facilitate developmental processes.

Assessing developmental processes

If the development of intellectual and affective processes is to be facilitated in students and given due prominence in the curriculum, such processes should be assessed. Self-assessment is very important but here the intention is to focus on a few practical ways in which teachers can help students in their written work. Beard and Hartley (1984) stress the importance of students developing sound study skills, and Gibbs (1981) provides a series of student-centred exercises to help improve study habits, note-taking, reading and writing skills. Habeshaw *et al.* (1989) describe a wide range of interesting exercises designed to help students with their studying. However, teachers also have an important role in developing students' intellectual skills by the tutorial support they give. The aim should be to extend the student's thinking and boost confidence when needed. Beard and Hartley (1984) discuss initial difficulties some students experience on beginning higher education. Thus some students believe that theories are 'true' and that authorities are beyond criticism. Teachers can help here by giving feedback in essays which is specific enough to pinpoint areas of difficulty. They can assist, too, by setting or negotiating written work and assignments which stimulate students and give them opportunities to develop and demonstrate their intellectual skills. Assessment criteria should include these skills. Valuing original thinking and independent comment are also important aspects of the teacher's role. This discussion has focused only on written work but a concern for general developmental processes should permeate the whole curriculum. The requirement that students have experience in a range of settings and with a variety of clients and patients offers further opportunities for such development.

Assessment in a range of settings and with a variety of clients and patients

The important point to note here is that in future pre-registration preparation the term 'practice settings' has wide connotations. Assessments will therefore take place in different settings and with a variety of clients and patients. Health education talks and caring for people at home or in clinics are all areas which could be assessed. Increasingly, then, the assessment of students is likely to become more complex and involve a wider range of assessors. However, profiling is a way of recording a student's progress in the practical and theoretical aspects of his or her work.

Profiles and profiling

Hitchcock (1986) defines a profile as 'a document which can record assessments of students across a wide range of abilities, including skills, attitudes, personal achievements, personal qualities and subject attainments'. The formative process is 'profiling' and the summative report 'the profile'. Profiling discussions can focus on the student's development in her theoretical and practical work and can involve self-assessment. The summative profile focuses on end achievements and can also include self-assessment and statements which have been negotiated between student and supervisor or teacher. Skelton (1989) discusses a continuous practical assessment scheme based on graded competencies in the context of profiling and profiles. Profile schemes enable assessment results to be reported in a way that focuses on individual development across a range of abilities, and they have a role in facilitating continuity through Common Foundation and branch programmes.

The issue of complexity in assessment schemes is, however, related to the question of evaluation, and this will be discussed in the context of current trends in nursing education.

Evaluation

Adelman and Alexander (1982) define educational evaluation as 'the making of judgements about the worth and effectiveness of educational intentions, processes and outcomes; about the relationships between these; about the resource, planning and implementation frameworks for such ventures'. The first phrase is important as it highlights the political nature of evaluation. For as Adelman and Alexander (1982) argue, the making of such judgements 'presupposes the existence of other, no doubt competing, values and judgements'. So it could be argued that teachers who hold different educational ideologies embodying conflicting beliefs about the nature of knowledge and justification for curricular decisions may emphasise different aspects of the evaluation process. They may, for example, differ in the importance they attach to the outcomes of learning as opposed to the experiences of learning, and in their views about the respective roles of teachers and students in the evaluation process. It is important, however, in relation to the four ideologies to ensure that evaluation strategies take into account the potential problems associated with each ideology. Beattie (1987) discusses some of these in the context of his Fourfold Curriculum. For example, he notes that with the 'basic skills' approach to curriculum, there is a danger that skills and practices may get out of date. The same can happen with the subject-mapping approach and indeed a curriculum can become packed too full of content. With the approach emphasising students' 'meaningful personal experiences' there is also the possibility that some learnings may not take place or that there are problems organising a range of different negotiated learning activities. A similar problem can occur with the 'agenda of cultural issues' approach.

The above points relate to evaluation as a means of course improvement, and they should be addressed as an integral part of an evaluation strategy, so as to avoid the dangers of 'curriculum inertia' (Lawton, 1983) or curriculum chaos! It is important, also, to examine whether the intentions of the institution and the course, as embodied in written philosophies, are actually reflected throughout the curriculum in action. These intentions will relate to course outcomes such as students' achievement of competencies, their understanding of knowledge content and the extent to which developmental processes have been facilitated. It is important to be alert for unintended or unexpected outcomes (Rowntree, 1985). Course intentions will also relate to the quality of the students' learning experiences. It is important to stress here that 'process approaches to evaluation (emphasising description and interpretation, dynamics and context) do not reject quantitative data or suggest that, in paying more attention to the process, outcomes be neglected' (Simons, 1987). Such comprehensive evaluation should involve students, teachers, and staff in practice settings, and scrutiny of material resources such as library books and films. A follow up evaluation six months or so after course completion can give useful feedback from recently qualified students.

However, much evaluation takes place informally at the micro level of the classroom or practice settings, and relates to what Rowntree (1985) calls the casual 'happen to notice' type of evaluation. Thus, it might be noticed that in their practical work students are not making theoretical links; or class attendance is dropping off; or even that colleagues are complaining about our students! (Rowntree, 1985). At this sort of informal level a useful and quick strategy is the 'graffiti technique'. This was used by Hitchens (1979) when she was faced by a large group of students who were continually late arriving and who talked and giggled in lectures. Discussion with them failed to resolve the problem so Hitchens offered them the opportunity to have ten minutes, without her present, in which they could write comments on three chalkboards. The headings for the boards were 'course content, method of presentation and class participation'. Under the third heading the class wrote statements about itself, all of which were negative. This opened the way for a discussion of themselves as a group and an increased self-awareness. The graffiti technique can be used, however, to get quick feedback at the end of a workshop or study day, and if a completely open-ended response is required, headings can be omitted.

Many of the evaluation strategies carried out with the intention of improving courses also assist in teacher development, and Chapter 8 includes a number of suggestions as to how teachers can evaluate the effectiveness of their teaching. However, not all evaluation is for 'insider' use. The ENB and academic bodies such as the Council for National Academic Awards (CNAA) require evidence of course evaluation, and the issue of Performance Indicators (PIs) in nursing education is being addressed as a high priority by the ENB.

Performance Indicators (PIs)

Balogh *et al.* (1989) produced a guide to assessing performance and quality in nursing and midwifery training institutions as part of an ENB funded project set up to examine the feasibility of developing PIs in such institutions. A key problem with PIs is knowing what they *are*. However, following their review of the literature, Balogh and Beattie (1988) suggest that most commentators would probably agree on three minimum properties of PIs. First, that they are 'numerical values which assess aspects of a system' (Balogh and Beattie, 1988). These values relate to aspects of the school's functioning such as the number of students starting, discontinuing and completing courses, and their employment destinations. The numbers of teachers in post, staff-student ratios, and the costs of the school would all be important data. A second property of PIs is that they are 'guides rather than absolute measures'. They *indicate* performance rather than *measure* it (Committee of Vice Chancellors and Principals, 1986). So, as Balogh *et al.* (1989) suggest, PIs 'raise questions'. A third property is that 'movement in indicators should be subject to unambiguous interpretation' (Best, 1986; cited by Balogh and Beattie, 1988). Three basic concepts associated with PIs are in the Audit Commission's 'three Es' model:

'Economy – how to obtain inputs of goods and services at the cheapest possible rate.
Efficiency – how much work it takes to do a given job; usually expressed as a ratio . .
Effectiveness – how well the job gets done according to the system's own criteria; success in achieving goals.'

(Balogh *et al.*, 1989)

PIs raise a number of issues. The idea of capturing the performance of an institution in stark numerical data seems unattractive but as Balogh *et al.* (1989) emphasise, *standards* and PIs should not be confused. The setting and maintenance of standards is essential but PIs themselves do not specify standards. A second issue relates to responsibility. In a climate of increasing financial stringency, professionals have to account for what they do in financial terms. Balogh *et al.* (1989) argue, however, the PIs can be a useful addition to an institution's repertoire of evaluation activities, and that in turn these existing strategies can be used to illuminate questions raised by PI data.

It is to stress the importance of standards, quality and professional judgement that Balogh *et al.* (1989) added a fourth 'E' to the Audit Commission's model: that of 'Ethics'. Ethical and political issues indeed permeate the whole evaluation process. As Adelman and Alexander (1982) point out, evaluation involves a number of decisions: about its purpose, focus and methods; the criteria to be used for judging worth and effectiveness; about who organises the evaluation, to whom the results are disseminated, and how the results will be used. With regard to the assessment of quality in nursing education Balogh *et al.* (1989) believe the best way forward is to use existing activities in schools, built upon if necessary. They argue that the ownership of results relating to performance and quality should remain firmly with the school. Simons (1987) indeed argues that schools need to formulate clear procedures governing access to and release of evaluation data.

Evaluation in nursing education is thus a complex area and is bound up with political and ethical issues. The same is also true of innovation in education and some of these issues will be discussed in the last part of this chapter.

Educational innovation

In relation to the literature on educational innovation House (1978) discusses the technological, political and cultural perspectives. The technological perspective is represented by writers such as Rogers and Shoemaker (1971); Havelock (1971); both cited by House (1978), and the emphasis in education was on large scale curriculum development projects planned centrally and disseminated to schools. Innovation was seen as a systematic and rational process, and as a 'good thing', hence the value laden terminology of 'laggards' (Rogers, 1962; cited by House, 1978).

In nursing education the technological perspective has much to offer, providing, as it does, clear guidelines for planning and implementing innovation. Docking (1987) and ENB (1987) both show how ideas from this perspective can be used to help plan and implement change in nursing education, and it will not therefore be examined further here. Instead the focus will be on the political and cultural perspectives.

House (1978) suggests that the earliest versions of the technological perspective which assumed consensus about innovation, gave way to a later version which accepted conflict as 'a price of progress'. Later, however, the interest in the innovation literature shifted to innovation as a political process. Here the emphasis is on value conflicts and opposing factions bargaining, negotiating and compromising. In the current context of nursing education, involving mergers of schools and links with higher education institutions, the political perspective may become increasingly relevant, and some of the issues involved will be explored a little further. Shaw (1975), for example, analysed the change process in an English College of Education and concluded that a continuous process of negotiation was at the centre of curriculum decision-making, and that the vital tasks for management were 'sustaining, facilitating and guiding this process and so far as possible increasing its effectiveness'. The groups involved were formally equal in status but there was a hierarchy of influence and power related to the size of departments and the spread of courses provided by each.

Squires (1987) discusses some of the difficulties which can arise when a field of study in higher education draws on several different disciplines, and he suggests that if one academic department is markedly larger or stronger than others, tensions can be created. Moreover, differences in teaching style which go unchallenged *within* a discipline become public in the context of interdisciplinary courses, and conflicts can arise over the relative importance of neatness of students' work, their referencing techniques, spelling and punctuality (Squires, 1987). A further issue relates to the distinction between theory and practice in courses. Squires (1987) suggests that this distinction affects the pecking order of subjects within higher education, the more theoretical ones being regarded as more difficult. According to this, nursing education could be seen as rather low down in the pecking order. Docking (1986), however, argues that a school of nursing needs to 'take on' the values and practices of higher education, such as scholarship and research, before moving into partnership, so that when this happens, it is on an equal footing. Staff development then is extremely important.

Understanding the politics of an institution is also a key element in negotiations. It is interesting to note that in one of the ENB's (1989b) case studies on higher education linkages, one of the polytechnic lecturers had initial difficulties in penetrating the nursing school because he did not understand the internal politics. Nevertheless, although a consideration of the political perspective sheds light on the complexity of the innovation process, it does not follow that conflict is always a dominant feature. One of the ENB's (1987) case studies suggests that the anger and frustration experienced by almost all the staff at the withdrawal of ENB course approval led to a channelling of energies to bring about the necessary changes.

House (1978) suggests that whereas the political perspective assumes that there is enough value consensus for the achievement of compromise, the cultural perspective assumes 'a more fragmented society, more value consensus within groups but less consensus among social groups so that groups must be regarded as subcultures'. Rudduck (1976; cited by House, 1978) discusses the culture of the innovation itself, the culture of the disseminating group and the culture of the classroom. The cultural perspective is particularly well discussed by Fullan (1982). Fullan argues that in planning change it is necessary to take into account its subjective and objective meanings. He discusses the subjective reality of educational change for teachers and notes its threatening and confusing nature and the tendency people have to try and change as little as possible. With regard to the objective reality of change, he suggests changes in practice can occur along three dimensions: new materials, new teaching approaches, and alteration of beliefs. Changes in beliefs and practices are the most difficult and are associated with much more fundamental change which therefore takes longer. When it comes to the outcome of change what really counts is the relationship between the objective reality of the new policies or curricular programmes, and the many subjective realities embedded in people's personal and organisational contexts (Fullan, 1982).

These three perspectives are evident in Chapter 9, in which the introduction of Information Technology in the curriculum is discussed. The perspectives are helpful in managing change because, as Atkin and House (1981) point out, they each focus on a different set of variables to explain the process of innovation, and they complement each other. One thing is certain: when people's educational ideologies are challenged change is more difficult and more profound. Some of the implications of this will be discussed in the last chapter when the theme of conflicting ideologies will be considered in the context of Beattie's (1987) dialectical curriculum. The dialectical approach is also explored in Chapter 2 in the context of planning the ethics component of a nursing curriculum.

A range of issues have been raised in this overview of key curricular elements and a number of these will be discussed in greater depth in ensuing chapters.

References

Adelman, C. and Alexander, R.J.   (1982).   *The Self-Evaluating Institution: Practice and Principles in the Management of Educational Change.* Methuen, London.

Allen, D.G. *et al.*   (1989).   Writing to learn: a reconceptualization of thinking and writing in the nursing curriculum. *Journal of Nursing Education*, **28(1)**, 6–11.

Allen M.   (1977).   *Evaluation of Educational Programmes in Nursing.* World Health Organisation, Geneva.

Allor, M.T.   (1983).   The community profile. *Journal of Nursing Education*, **22(1)**, 12–17.

Archer, T. (1988). Student power. *Nursing Times and Nursing Mirror*, **84(42)**, 49–51.

Atkin, J.M. and House, E.R. (1981). The federal role in curriculum development, 1950–1980. *Educational Evaluation and Policy Analysis*, **3(5)**, 5–36.

Balogh, R. and Beattie, A. (1988). *Performance Indicators in Nursing Education: Final Report on a Feasibility Study carried out for the English National Board for Nursing, Midwifery and Health Visiting.* Institute of Education, University of London.

Balogh, R. *et al.* (1989). *Figuring out Performance: A Guide to Assessing Performance and Quality in Nursing and Midwifery Training Institutions.* English National Board for Nursing, Midwifery and Health Visiting, London.

Beard, R.M. and Hartley, J. (1984). *Teaching and Learning in Higher Education.* Fourth edition. Harper and Row, London.

Beattie, A. (1987). Making a curriculum work. In *The Curriculum in Nursing Education*, P. Allan and M. Jolley (Eds), pp. 15–34. Croom Helm, London.

Blenkin, G.M. and Kelly, A.V. (1987). *The Primary Curriculum: A Process Approach to Curriculum Planning.* Second edition. Harper and Row, London.

Brookfield, S.D. (1987) *Developing Critical Thinkers: Challenging Adults to Explore Alternative Ways of Thinking and Acting.* Open University Press, Milton Keynes.

Bruner, J.S. (1966). *Toward a Theory of Instruction.* Belknap Press for Harvard University Press, Cambridge, Massachusetts.

Bruner, J.S. (1977). *The Process of Education.* Second edition. Harvard University Press, Cambridge, Massachusetts.

Burnard, P. (1988). The journal as an assessment and evaluation tool in nurse education. *Nurse Education Today*, **8(2)**, 105–7.

Carlisle, D. (1989). Defending the ozone. *Nursing Standard*, **3(40)**, 14–16.

Committee of Vice Chancellors and Principals (1986). *Performance Indicators in Universities. A first statement by a joint C.U.C.P./U.G.C. working group.* CUCP, London.

Cooper, S.S. (1986). Teaching tips. Advice columns as a teaching tool. *Journal of Continuing Education in Nursing*, **17(5)**, 181.

Curriculum Development Centre (1982). Core curriculum for Australian schools. In *Challenge and Change in the Curriculum*. T. Horton and P. Raggatt (Eds), pp. 104–17. Hodder & Stoughton in association with the Open University, Sevenoaks.

Currie, E. and Maynard, A. (1989). *The Economics of Hospital Acquired Infection.* Centre for Health Economics, University of York. (Discussion Paper 56.)

de Tornyay, R. and Thompson, M.A. (1987). *Strategies for Teaching Nursing.* Third edition. Wiley, New York.

Department of Health (1990). *Health Care Assistants.* DOH, London. [EL(MB) 90/5].

Dewey, J. (1916). *Democracy and Education.* The Free Press, New York.

Dobson, S. (1986). Ethnography: a tool for learning. *Nurse Education Today*, **6(2)**, 76–9.

Docking, S. (1986). *Towards a Climate of Creativity: A Strategy for Innovation in One School of Nursing. King's Fund Conference: Blueprint for the Future?* King's Fund Centre, London.

Docking, S.   (1987).   Curriculum innovation. In *The Curriculum in Nursing Education*, P. Allan and M. Jolley (Eds), pp. 149–63. Croom Helm, London.

Eisner, E.W.   (1975).   Instructional and expressive objectives. In *Curriculum Design*, M. Golby *et al.* (Eds), pp. 351–4. Croom Helm in association with the Open University Press, London.

Eisner, E.W.   (1985).   *The Educational Imagination: On the Design and Evaluation of School Programs.* Second edition. Macmillan, New York.

English National Board for Nursing, Midwifery and Health Visiting (1985). *Professional Education/Training Courses: Consultation Paper.* ENB, London.

English National Board for Nursing, Midwifery and Health
   Visiting   (1987).   *Managing Change in Nursing Education – Section 3: The process of innovation.* ENB, London.

English National Board for Nursing, Midwifery and Health
   Visiting   (1989a).   *Health Promotion in Primary Health Care: An Introduction. An Open Learning Package for Practice Nurses.* ENB, London.

English National Board for Nursing, Midwifery and Health
   Visiting   (1989b).   *Managing Change in Nursing Education – Section 1: Tackling organisational change.* ENB, London.

English National Board for Nursing, Midwifery and Health
   Visiting   (1989c).   *Project 2000 – 'A New Preparation for Practice'. Guidelines and Criteria for Course Development and the Formation of Collaborative Links between Approved Training Institutions within the National Health Service and Centres of Higher Education.* ENB, London.

Ewan, C. and White, R.   (1984).   *Teaching Nursing: A Self-Instructional Handbook.* Croom Helm, London.

Feinmann, J. (1989). Going for green. *Nursing Times and Nursing Mirror*, **85(14)**, 16, 18.

Fullan, M.   (1982).   *The Meaning of Educational Change.* Teachers College Press, Columbia University, New York.

Gibbs, G.   (1981).   *Teaching Students to Learn.* Open University, Milton Keynes.

Gilling, C.M.   (1989).   A common core curriculum for nurses, midwives and health visitors. *Nurse Education Today*, **9(2)**, 82–92.

Habeshaw, T. *et al.*   (1989).   *53 Interesting Ways of Helping Your Students to Study.* Second edition. Technical and Educational Services, Bristol.

Hahnemann, B.K.   (1986).   Journal writing: a key to promoting critical thinking in nursing students. *Journal of Nursing Education*, **25(5)**, 213–15.

Hamilton, D. *et al.* (Eds)   (1977).   The objectives model revisited: editors' introduction. In *Beyond the Numbers Game*, D. Hamilton *et al.* (Eds) pp. 25–8. Macmillan Education, Basingstoke.

Henderson, V.A.   (1989).   Countdown to 2000: a major international conference for the primary health care team, 21–23 September 1987, London. Conference report. *Journal of Advanced Nursing*, **14(1)**, 81–5.

Heron, J.   (1988).   Assessment revisited. In *Developing Student Autonomy in Learning*, D. Boud (Ed.). Second edition. pp. 77–90. Kogan Page, London.

Hirst, P.H. and Peters, R.S.   (1970).   *The Logic of Education.* Routledge and Kegan Paul, London.

Hirst, P.H. (1974). *Knowledge and the Curriculum.* Routledge and Kegan Paul, London.
Hitchcock, G. (1986). *Profiles and Profiling: a practical introduction.* Longman, Harlow.
Hitchens, E.W. (1979). Evaluation: the graffiti technique. *Journal of Nursing Education,* **18(3)**, 46–7.
Holly, M.L. and McLoughlin, C.S. (1989). Professional development and journal writing. In *Perspectives on Teacher Professional Development,* M.L. Holly and C.S. McLoughlin (Eds), pp. 259–83. The Falmer Press, London.
House, E.R. (1978). Technology versus craft: a ten year perspective on innovation. In *New Directions in Curriculum Studies,* P.H. Taylor (Ed.), pp. 137–51. Falmer Press, Lewes.
Howden, C. and Baggaley, S. (1989). Learning from the experts. *Nursing Times and Nursing Mirror,* **85(25)**, 42–4.
Jarvis, P. (1983). *Professional Education.* Croom Helm, London.
Kelly, A.V. (1986). *Knowledge and Curriculum Planning.* Harper and Row, London.
Kelly, A.V. (1989). *The Curriculum. Theory and Practice.* Third edition. Paul Chapman, London.
Kenworthy, N. and Nicklin, P. (1989). *Teaching and Assessing in Nursing Practice: An Experiential Approach.* Scutari Press, London.
Knowles, M. (1978). *The Adult Learner: a Neglected Species.* Gulf Publishing Co., Houston, Texas.
Lantz, J.M. and Meyers, G.D. (1986). Critical thinking through writing: using personification to teach pharmacodynamics. *Journal of Nursing Education,* **25(2)**, 64–6.
Lawton, D. (1981). *An Introduction to Teaching and Learning.* Hodder & Stoughton, London.
Lawton, D. (1983). *Curriculum Studies and Educational Planning.* Hodder & Stoughton, London.
Lyall, J. (1989). Foreign bodies. *Nursing Times and Nursing Mirror,* **85(25)**, 16–17.
Martin, D. (1989). Market Forces. *Nursing Standard,* **3(33)**, **34–5.**
McFarlane, J. (1989). Whitewashing the past. *Nursing Times and Nursing Mirror,* **85(14)**, 46–7.
National Council for Vocational Qualifications (1987). *The National Vocational Qualification Framework.* NCVQ, London.
National Council for Vocational Qualifications (n.d.). *The National Council for Vocational Qualifications in England, Wales and Northern Ireland. Its Purposes and Aims.* HMSO, London.
Oliver, R. (1988). Out and about. *Nursing Times and Nursing Mirror,* **84(28)**, 63–4.
Orr, J. (1988). Designing the way forward. *Nursing Times and Nursing Mirror,* **84(37)**, 46–7.
Pearce, C. (1988). The nursing workforce. *Senior Nurse,* **8(3)**, 25–7.
Peters, R.S. (1966). *Ethics and Education.* Allen and Unwin, London.
Peters, R.S. (1981). *Essays on Educators.* Allen and Unwin, London.
Porter, A. (Ed.) (1983). *Teaching Political Literacy.* Institute of Education, University of London. (Bedford Way Paper 16.)

Rogers, C. (1983). *Freedom to Learn for the 80's.* Charles E. Merrill, Columbus, Ohio.

Rowntree, D. (1982). *Educational Technology In Curriculum Development.* Second edition. Harper and Row, London.

Rowntree, D. (1985). *Developing Courses for Students.* Harper and Row, London.

Rowntree, D. (1987). *Assessing Students: How Shall We Know Them?* Second edition. Kogan Page, London.

Royal College of Nursing of the United Kingdom (1989). *Standards of Care for Health Visiting.* Scutari Press, Harrow. (RCN Standards of Care Project.)

Schools Council (1976). *Schools Council History 13–16 Project: What is History? Teachers' Guide.* Holmes McDougall, Edinburgh.

Scrimshaw, P. (1983). *Unit 2 Educational ideologies. Educational Studies: A Second Level Course E204 Purpose and Planning in the Curriculum, Block 1 Society, the education system and the curriculum.* Open University, Milton Keynes.

Shaw, K.E. (1975). Negotiating curriculum change in a College of Education. In *Case Studies in Curriculum Change*, W.A. Reid and D.F. Walker (Eds), pp. 54–90. Routledge and Kegan Paul, London.

Simons, H. (1987). *Getting to Know Schools in a Democracy: The Politics and Process of Evaluation.* The Falmer Press, London.

Skelton, G.M. (1989). Assessment and profiling of clinical performance. In *Teaching and Assessing in Clinical Nursing Practice*, P.L. Bradshaw (Ed.), pp. 160–74. Prentice Hall, New York.

Skilbeck, M. (1975). The school and cultural development. In *Curriculum Design*, M. Golby *et al.* (Eds), pp. 27–35. Croom Helm in association with the Open University, London.

Skilbeck, M. (1982a). Three educational ideologies. In *Challenge and Change in the Curriculum*, T. Horton and P. Raggatt (Eds), pp. 7–18. Hodder & Stoughton in association with the Open University, Sevenoaks.

Skilbeck, M. (1982b). School-based curriculum development. In *Planning in the Curriculum*, V. Lee and D. Zeldin (Eds), pp. 18–34. Hodder & Stoughton in association with the Open University, Sevenoaks.

Skilbeck, M. (1984). *School-based Curriculum Development.* Harper and Row, London.

Skilbeck, M. (1985). *A Core Curriculum for the Common School.* Second edition. Institute of Education, University of London.

Sobralske, M.C. (1989). Students can enhance writing skills while promoting health. *Nurse Educator*, **14(1)**, 38–9.

Sockett, H. (1976a). Unit 16 Approaches to curriculum planning I. In *Rationality and Artistry. Educational Studies: A Second Level Course E203 Curriculum Design and Development*, pp. 3–31. Open University, Milton Keynes.

Sockett, H. (1976b). *Designing the Curriculum.* Open Books, London.

Squires, G. (1987). *The Curriculum Beyond School.* Hodder & Stoughton, London.

Steinaker, N.W. and Bell, M.R. (1979). *The Experiential Taxonomy: A New Approach to Teaching and Learning.* Academic Press, New York.

Stenhouse, L. (1975). *An Introduction to Curriculum Research and Development.* Heinemann, London.

Stenhouse, L. (1985). The process model in action: the Humanities Curriculum Project. In *Research as a Basis for Teaching. Readings from the work of Lawrence Stenhouse*, J. Rudduck and D. Hopkins, (Eds), pp. 89–91. Heinemann Educational, London.

Taylor, P.H. and Richards, C.M. (1985). *An Introduction to Curriculum Studies*. Second edition. NFER – Nelson, Windsor.

Tyler, R.W. (1949). *Basic Principles of Curriculum and Instruction*. University of Chicago Press, Chicago.

United Kingdom Central Council for Nursing, Midwifery and Health Visiting (1985). *Project 2000: Facing the Future, Project Paper 6*. UKCC, London.

United Kingdom Central Council for Nursing, Midwifery and Health Visiting (1986). *Project 2000: A New Preparation for Practice*. UKCC, London.

United Kingdom Central Council for Nursing, Midwifery and Health Visiting (1988). *UKCC's Proposed Rules for the Standard, Kind and Content of Future Pre- Registration Nursing Education. Consultation Paper*. September. UKCC, London.

Walsh, M. (1989). Clean air lobby. *Nursing Standard*, **3(45)**, 34–5.

Weil, S. (1952). *The Need for Roots. Prelude to a Declaration of Duties towards Mankind*. Routledge and Kegan Paul, London.

Wheeler, D.K. (1967). *Curriculum Process*. Hodder & Stoughton, London.

Whitehead, M. (1988). The health divide. In *Inequalities in Health*, P. Townsend *et al.* (Eds), pp. 215–356. Penguin, London.

Wysocki, R. (1980). Evaluation of student clinical performance. *Australian Nurses' Journal*, **10(5)**, 42–3.

2 Planning the ethics component of a curriculum

Sally Glen

Introduction

'Education is a view of the world from the point of view of learning to live in that world. Its horizons and its limitations are close to the society of which it is part'

(Priestley, 1987)

Nursing ethics might be described as a reflection of the profession's morality, or 'moral view of the world'. However, this would be misguided. Nursing ethics is a part of general morality or the general moral 'view of the world', and it is for this reason that situational analysis (Tyler, 1949; Skilbeck, 1984) is an appropriate prerequisite to planning and developing the ethics component of a Common Foundation Programme and branch programmes for Project 2000 (United Kingdom Central Council for Nursing, Midwifery and Health Visiting (UKCC), 1986).

This chapter begins by discussing the need for a flexible approach to curriculum models, and by outlining some of the external and internal factors which form a context for planning the ethics component of a Common Foundation Programme. Following this the notion of 'situational analysis' is used to explore how the hidden curriculum and nursing educational ideologies such as 'autonomy' add to the complexity of planning the ethics components of a curriculum. Finally, a dialectical approach to curriculum planning in this area is proposed and worked examples are included to show how theoretical principles could be put into practice.

Curriculum planning: the importance of context

How does one begin to plan and develop the ethics component of a Common Foundation or branch programme? As the term 'situational analysis' implies, the answer has everything to do with the specific college of nursing and its specific context; with a recognition that each school/college of nursing is unique by virtue of its history, type or location. (This point is discussed further in Chapter 10.) It is important to emphasise, therefore, that the broad framework outlined in this chapter must be *tested in practice* by teacher practitioners, and modified accordingly. Nurse teachers should be guided, not led by the literature. This suggests a shift away from the notion of curriculum theory being applied to curriculum practice. Instead, the relationship between theory

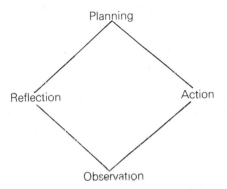

Fig. 2.1 The curriculum planning and development process underpinned by the action-research cycle.

and practice might be conceptualised as cyclical (Fig. 2.1). Consequently, curriculum is inextricably linked with the experience of educational practice. Practice and theory are a seamless web. Underpinning the approach to curriculum planning and development advocated in this chapter, therefore, are three notions: that literature on the curriculum should guide rather than lead nurse teachers; that the relationship between theory and practice is cyclical; and that curriculum planning takes place in unique contexts. The emphasis on unique contextual factors in planning is a key feature of Skilbeck's (1984) situational analysis model.

Skilbeck's situational analysis model

Skilbeck's (1984) 'situational analysis' emphasises the context within which a curriculum exists, including the social atmosphere and existing relationships. The 'Situational Analysis–Goals Definition–Curriculum Development–Evaluation Model' (Fig. 2.2) was originally designed to guide primary and secondary school teachers, but it lends itself to adaptation and indeed Skilbeck suggests that it is applicable to the whole range of curriculum projects. Thus it could guide the planning of large scale national curriculum innovations as well as smaller and more modest innovations within a faculty or department of a college

Analyse the situation

Define the objectives

Design the teaching-learning programme

Interpret and implement the programme

Assess and Evaluate

Fig. 2.2 The Situational Analysis–Goals Definition–Curriculum Development–Evaluation Model (from Skilbeck, 1984).

of nursing. In considering the flexibility of his approach it is interesting to note that Skilbeck (1984) has moved away from the concept of curriculum model, with its connotation of 'blue-print', to that of 'design brief'. He underlines the flexibility of the concept of 'design' as opposed to 'model', when he suggests that

'designs for human action, in use, become quite varied and may lose much of their original sharpness. Recognition of this fact is a necessary part of understanding curriculum implementation; it is a mark of our awareness that curriculum change is a social and environmental affair in which human relations, organisational factors and institutional politics all play their part.'

(Skilbeck, 1984)

This shift in thinking about the relationship between a curriculum model and a design brief, and that between curriculum theory and educational practice is not merely intellectual, it is also profoundly political. Skilbeck is underlining the fact that curriculum planning and development is a sociopolitical affair.

Returning specifically to planning of an ethics component of the curriculum, the loose framework, outlined in Fig. 2.2, might be used as a guide to collaborative, structured decision-making. It is important, however, that the following points are considered:

(i)   The 'design brief' should be seen as a sequence of problematic issues to be resolved in practice, rather than as a framework for legitimation of curriculum ideas. If the curriculum planning and development process is not seen in this way, complex issues may be simplified to a misleading degree. This leads to criticisms of the approach being a wooden and technical model of curriculum development (Carr and Kemmis, 1986).

(ii)   Decisions may oscillate rather than progress; the framework does not imply step-by-step progression. For example, objectives set early on should be revisited and may need progressive modification as the educational process develops.

(iii)   The design brief offers a challenge to unease and ambivalence

about objectives and Skilbeck's (1984) reappraisal of the appropriateness of objectives, as an approach to curriculum planning and development, has much to recommend to nurse teachers. It could be argued that
general objectives and expressive activities and outcomes (discussed
in Chapter 1) have a place in planning the ethics component of a
curriculum.

Situational analysis: external and internal factors

As a key part of the curriculum planning process Skilbeck (1984)
recommends carrying out an external and internal situational analysis.
Below are examples of external and internal factors which form the
context of the ethics component of a Common Foundation Programme.

External factors

The external factors, which nurse teachers might consider, include the
following.

- The UKCC's Project 2000 intention that education should facilitate the development of a thoughtful nurse with the knowledge
  and experience to form her own judgements at work (UKCC,
  1986).

- The English National Board for Nursing, Midwifery and Health
  Visiting (ENB) learning outcomes, which include 'understanding of
  the ethics of the nursing profession and the responsibilities which
  these impose on the nurse's professional practice' (ENB, 1989).

- Greater acknowledgement of the pluralistic nature of society and
  the 'open and loaded' (Walsh, 1988) nature of what constitutes
  'health'.

- The movement towards improving communication between different sections of the National Health Service coupled with an examination of old hierarchies (Department of Health and Social Security
  Community Nursing Review, 1986).

- The tensions and contradictions inherent in claiming professional
  autonomy for primary nurses within bureaucratic organisational
  structures, such as hospitals (Bowers, 1989).

- The emergence of new practice paradigms that make it necessary
  for nurses to take responsibility for health education and develop
  partnership, or fiduciary relationships with clients and patients
  (Wilson-Barnett, 1989). Project 2000 is not just an exercise in education reform. It is a change in the philosophy of health care.

- Increasing interest in the ideas of 'holism' and holistic health care,
  making it possible and desirable for primary nurses to be seen as
  practitioners in their own right.

- The conflict between nursing's proclaimed humanistic ethics and the ascendency of managerial and business ethics (Crowley, 1989a).

Finally, but by no means least significantly, the moral education of nurses raises significant questions about the sort of health care service one wishes to foster and the kind of health care professional one wishes to practise within that service. There are, however, large inter/intra professional and consumer disagreements over the function and role of the National Health Service and thus over what constitutes the 'virtuous' nurse.

Internal Factors

Internal factors that might be considered include the following.

- The specific community profile of the college/clinical environment.

- The educational philosophy underpinning the whole curriculum.

- The need for the integration of ethics throughout the curriculum to be made more explicit.

- The human resources ('teacher' values, skills and knowledge) and the material resources available to plan, develop, teach and evaluate this component of the curriculum.

- Students' needs and interests as negotiated continuously throughout the course.

The important point here is that curriculum planners and developers never start with a 'carte blanche'. As Handy (1984) notes in his analysis of schools as organisations: 'Organisations are to some extent stuck with their past, with their reputation, the kinds of people they hired years ago, their site and their traditions'. Consequently, schools of nursing vary very significantly in terms of what Handy has called their 'culture'. This culture is related to the educational philosophy of the school/college and the course aims, and both of these should be made explicit. The ethics component of the Common Foundation or branch programme, for example, should be based upon certain characteristics which the individual school/college of nursing has decided define the educated nurse. For example, the central aim of the St. Mary's School of Nursing three year diploma course is '... to equip reflective professionals with a sound educational base in order to meet the present and future health care needs of society'. These are professionals who 'are able and willing to be the agents of and respondents to change, in an environment of greater professional unity', and who can 'offer constructive nursing participation with other members of the multidisciplinary health care team, in overall health policy formulation, implementation and evaluation' (St. Mary's School of Nursing, 1989).

The school's/college's definition of an educated nurse could be both aspired to by students, and one which they could identify as already being partly achieved.

The curriculum as a whole should also be based on an explicit educational philosophy. For example, the St. Mary's School of Nursing philosophy for the Common Foundation Programme includes this statement:

'.... The Educational ethos needs to be such that it is reflective of, and supportive towards, forms of student development, such as critical analytical skills. Traditional 'School of Nursing' structures which depend on hierarchical arrangements of power and status, are clearly incompatible with values associated with holism. Partnership, co-ownership, self-directedness, and autonomy are ways of fostering experiential learning of the kind of values which will underpin the approach of professional practice promoted by the UKCC'.

(St Mary's School of Nursing, 1989)

The hidden curriculum

Situational analysis underlines the social context and relationships within which a curriculum exists and these are also constituent components of the hidden curriculum. The hidden curriculum is a concept developed in general education (Bowles and Gintis, 1976; Apple, 1979) which refers to the values 'hidden' in the relationships, structures and formal curriculum of the school or college. Values are implicit in, and conveyed through, the choice of certain activities rather than others, the opinions expressed (Davis, 1989), the various stable procedures through which business is conducted towards the individual, the attitude of teacher to teacher, teacher to student (Crowley, 1989b), student to student and towards the community as whole.

In planning the ethics component of a curriculum teachers cannot afford to ignore Williams' (1987) comment that 'One of the most important facts about morality is its concrete social reality – the whole reality of ethics resides in social practices and institutions.' The management and organisational structures of colleges/schools of nursing and clinical environments form part of the hidden curriculum for nurse teachers, nurse practitioners and students (Glen, 1989) but to date few studies in nursing education have focused on this hidden curriculum. Three studies, however, are of particular relevance: Melia (1981), Clinton (1981) and Treacy (1987). Treacy asserts that her work 'identifies a hidden curriculum in the hospital training schools studied. Accounts suggest that student nurses experience powerlessness, uncertainty and depersonalisation; this experience is conceptualised as "pipeline status". It is suggested that this results in a compliance and a conformity on the part of individuals as they depend on existing structures and routines to "get by"'. Feminists have also documented the psychological costs of working within hierarchical/bureaucratic structures. Ferguson (1984), for example, describes 'the personal consequences of a powerless, non-participatory existence'.

There is no doubt that moral development, within the context of professional practice, should be a major concern for nurse teachers. However, it is mistaken to conclude that the way of translating this concern into curriculum terms is to put another subject, namely ethics, on the timetable. Curriculum development, in this area, must at least begin with an attempt to make explicit the 'hidden' values and assumptions implicit in the college/school of nursing and clinical environment, and to subject them to analysis and criticism. There are significant questions to be asked, for example, about the articulated aims of nursing education.

The author reviewed the philosophies of education pertaining to approximately ten different colleges/schools of nursing (Glen, 1988). The most striking commonality was that much of nursing education appears to be fuelled by the notion of developing autonomy in students. Furthermore, the working vocabulary of nurse teachers was replete with concepts such as 'individual development', 'personal growth', 'autonomy' and 'self-direction', which can all be prefaced with the word 'individual'. This suggests that nursing education is not primarily concerned with creating a certain kind of health care service, sensitive to the health care needs of society, but rather, its primary duty is the promotion of the autonomous individual. However, analysis of the conceptual characteristics associated with autonomy suggests that needs may be conceptualised in terms which fail to take into account the notion of human interdependence. Yet ironically 'interdependence' may be a key concept for nursing in the 'Year 2000'. It should be stressed that the intention is not to claim that this concern with the individual student nurse's personal, social and moral development is entirely misguided. Rather it is to suggest that the individual and the social are both interdependent concepts, and yet potentially in conflict with one another. The art consists in holding these two elements in some kind of balance, in ensuring that the conflict between the two is held in a constructive tension (Hargreaves, 1980).

The importance of the concept 'interdependence' in nursing is discussed by Bergman (1976) who, debating the issue of evolving ethical concepts for nursing, suggested that there is a new ethic of personal responsibility for nursing practice: one of social commitment and accountability. She is referring to a situation where an individual presents to others, for scrutiny, information relating to the actions she or he has taken. Bergman (1976) writes: '. . . it is an ethic from dependence to independence to interdependence from separateness towards togetherness with colleagues and community.' The concept of autonomy, on the other hand, is set within the structure of nursing education's social and educational values, but its conceptual characteristics do not have any necessary implications for the development of a positive commitment to others in terms of care, concern and compassion. Therefore, in advocating the development of autonomy as one of the characteristics of an 'ideal nurse', teachers are forced to adopt a somewhat paradoxical position and certainly one that is incongruent with education for health care. However, a concern to stress the capacities for caring and empathy for others, which are pivotal to education for a caring profession, may lead to the conceptualising of such capacities in terms which seem to leave little space for the needs of the individual self – hence the need to maintain a constructive tension between the individual and the social.

The point that is being made is that any theorising applicable to the ethics component of the nursing curriculum must recognise the extent to which the identity of individuals is constituted in something which they and their clients and patients inherit. As Ward (1983) notes: 'We are children of our time and culture and not dispassionate choosers of our destiny.' It is also important for students to appreciate that obligations and values are defined by their roles as nurses. For this reason it is misguided for nurse teachers to propagate the notion of a free market of ideas in which 'consumers' will 'buy' the best, and therefore choose freely. It also undervalues social obligations, and is therefore a highly political stance. The irony of such an approach to the moral education of student nurses, fuelled by the notion of autonomy as an ideal, is that it can breed a sort of arrogance, which rejects tradition just because it is old and unfashionable. Spickerman (1988), however, suggests that student nurses should be educated to work within a matrix of conformity to a certain tradition, and criticism of that tradition, and Haydon (1987) argues that without a certain background of tradition there can be no such thing as the rational, autonomous moral agent. Nurse teachers must, therefore, seek a curriculum framework which stresses the values of accepting traditions of thought and perception, and understanding and valuing them sympathetically. What is required is a creative reshaping of such traditions, rather than their outright rejection, and an acknowledgement that all of us are rooted in traditions of thought.

Finally, to conclude this section it is suggested that the primary aim of every school/college of nursing must be the enhancement of caring. But how does one operationalise this abstract concept in the context of nursing education? (Hedin and Donovan, 1989). In tackling this problem curriculum planners might find it helpful to consider the practical implications of the following statements.

- There is an interdependence between the style of management of an institution and the style of care it produces (Kohnke, 1982).

- Changing nursing practice paradigms make varied demands on nurses. In turn, nurses themselves need varied support such as effective occupational health departments, counselling services, support groups, mentoring (Palmer, 1987; Burnard, 1988; Laurent, 1988; Morris *et al.*, (1988) and preceptor relationships (Shamian and Inhaber, 1985; Myrick, 1988).

• If nursing is a profession in transition then hopefully the transitional process will be punctuated with much critical self-examination of taken-for-granted beliefs, ideologies and clichés (Glen, 1988; Wilson-Barnett, 1988).

Teaching ethics: some theoretical perspectives

In Aldous Huxley's (1932) novel *Brave New World* the Director of Hatcheries and Conditioning argued that moral education 'Ought never, in any circumstances to be rational'. If there is anything common to the contemporary approaches to moral education, within the context of nursing education, it is an indignant and justifiably acrimonious opposition to any such point of view. However, the argument that will be developed in this section is that curricular approaches can be criticised for being too rational or rather, more correctly, their focus reflects a heavily cognitive approach.

Hide (1980) based her earlier work on Wilson (1969) who talks in terms of equipping students with the concepts to engage in autonomous moral thinking. Clay *et al.* (1983) looked to Fenton and Kohlberg's (1976) earlier work. They argued that by exposing students to *dilemmas*, in a systematic and regular way, and by encouraging them in groups to discuss the appropriate action and the reasons for achieving that action, a teacher could accomplish a measurable development in the student's moral reasoning. The theory underpinning this approach (i.e. group discussion of ethical dilemmas) was initially developed by Piaget, and subsequently in considerable detail by Kohlberg, who has empirically identified five stages of moral reasoning (Piaget, 1932; Kohlberg, 1976; cited by Weinreich-Haste, 1987; Kohlberg *et al.*, 1983).

Approaches to the ethics component of nursing curricula tend to be 'Kohlbergian' (Hide, 1987); in other words there is an emphasis on the presentation of hypothetical moral dilemmas in an effort to stimulate moral development from a cognitive perspective. Consequently many ethics curricula can be criticised because they have largely concentrated on the process of developing critical thinking and their conception of the rational enterprise and the moral life is thus one-sided and incomplete. This emphasis gives contemporary nursing ethics a mathematical appearance. Even though philosophers and curriculum planners have recognised the difference between 'pure' or logical reason and 'practical' or moral reason, ethical argumentation in nursing education had frequently proceeded as if it were governed by the logical necessity characteristic of geometry. Moral decisions are, after all, made in real situations; they are qualitatively different from the solutions of geometry problems. Arranging principles hierarchically, and deriving conclusions logically, is peripheral to, or even alien to many problems in nursing. Most of our recognisable moral life, indeed, is conducted in a relatively unreflective and spontaneous way. We appraise people as kind, gentle or modest, not because they have the right kind of principles but because they feel about people and situations in a certain sort of way.

Dykstra (1981) argues that some form of vision is necessary for any proper account of morality. He suggests that what we really mean when we speak of a person's moral life is 'their ongoing quality of life, their total vision of life'. It is a vision that is possibly required by student nurses if they are to develop into 'Productive Rule Breakers' – a term coined by Prophit (1987). Feelings, needs, impressions and a sense of personal ideal are required, rather than the application of principles. Nurse teachers concerned with developing the ethics component of the nursing curriculum must acknowledge that reason describes a human power far beyond the capacity for making of numbers and measures. Reason does not merely refer to logical techniques or organised rational sifting. It has very little to do with the completed understanding implied in solving problems. It has to do with the unique relationship the nurse experiences between him or herself and his or her client, whose values, whose meaning, he or she is trying to absorb more fully. It requires that nurses use their talents and intellectual disciplines and capacities to analyse, but always implicit in the situation is the realisation that there is no finally complete grasp of meaning.

Another approach, commonly used in nursing education, is *values clarification*. Clamp (1984) looked to Raths *et al.* (1966) and Simon (1972) who are associated with values clarification and who represent one philosophical position which casts doubt upon objectivity. Indeed, this scepticism permeates much educational thinking about moral development. The premise underpinning this approach is that students ought to be free to choose and to create their own values. The nurse teacher's role is to help students to clarify their values and to make up their own minds. There are therefore certain values that are presupposed here and now to be freely chosen, namely those of freedom to choose. The question of how free the student is to choose has been discussed earlier in this chapter.

To identify values clarification with moral education would be wrong. It would however be equally wrong to dismiss it and its very practical teaching strategies. Personal growth and the achievement of autonomy in a more acceptable sense, does require a clarification of where one stands on various issues and a clarification too of the alternative solutions to the moral issues one is confronted with. Any teaching strategy that helps with this is welcomed, so long as it does not give the impression that there is no context to morality which needs to be learnt and to be respected. Lovin (1988), however, argues that rather than encouraging students simply to clarify their values, teachers should foster the articulation of values. By this he has in mind a process which will involve students in a critical examination of values in the light of the traditions of reflection on them and which will serve as a preparation for the wider public discussion of values. Lovin suggests that there are 'some positions that a teacher can safely eliminate as contenders in reasonable public discussion'. However, what is a reasonable position is not likely to be an uncontentious matter.

Approaches to the teaching of ethics, therefore, tend to be reductionist. Morality is equated with decision-making, decision-making is then viewed as reasoning, and reasoning is conceived of as judging, with dilemmas in conflict situations assumed to be the proper object of that activity. Paradoxically, in the context of the student's daily life, major moral dilemmas are the exception, not the rule. That is not to say that students never confront dilemmas, but moral life is not reducible to a series of dilemmas, nor is it comprised mainly of them. Neither is the resolution of conflict, whether between opposing parties to dispute, between one's own desired and moral principles or between competing principles, the only or even the most important element of moral thought and action. It is interesting, though, that according to Schröck (1980) '. . . most of the writings, meetings, discussions, study days and slots in the nursing student's timetable which are devoted at least occasionally to 'moral dilemmas in nursing' by and large use examples of experience and events which cannot in any sense be described as everyday happenings'. Although this was written ten years ago, it is probably still applicable today in many schools of nursing.

As a concluding remark to this section, it is suggested that in defining the morally educated nurse as one possessing rational mind, and in construing this in narrow, intellectualistic terms, feelings and emotions and other so-called non-cognitive states and processes of the individual are all but ignored. Nursing education has therefore tended to emulate a model of moral education which is neither tolerant nor generous, and which is incongruent with the raison d'être of education for health care. However, when qualities such as care, concern and compassion are included in the nurse teacher's description of the educational ideal, then the framework underpinning the ethics component of the curriculum must be vitally transformed.

In the next section a curriculum structure is outlined in which affectivity is not in opposition with reason, nor care with justice. It is an attempt to transcend dualistic and polarised curricular frameworks which dichotomise individual and society, subject and object, emotions and reason, thought and action.

Planning the ethics component of the curriculum: a dialectical framework

Inherent in the dialectical approach to curriculum planning is the idea that aspects of different theories can be deliberately drawn upon in the development of a single programme. The dialectical approach is discussed further in Chapter 10 of this book. Such an approach, of course, is not without its own hazards. One major consideration must be to try to ensure maximum compatibility among the various theoretical elements going to make the whole. Nevertheless, when qualities such as care, concern, compassion, rights and justice are included in the nurse teacher's description of the educational ideal, the framework underpinning the ethics component of the curriculum must be a dialectical framework. Education for health care must be concerned with both relationship-orientated qualities and reasoning abilities.

In formulating a dialectical framework for the ethics component of a curriculum, the works of Rest (1983) and Habermas (1978) have much to offer nurse teachers. Rest (1983) identifies four different components of morality:

— Moral reasoning
— Ethical sensitivity
— Action related to a moral position
— Commitment to a moral stance

The first of these, namely moral reasoning, is an essentially cognitive component of morality; it is concerned with a rational form of moral decision-making. 'Ethical sensitivity' can be interpreted as the capacity to recognise and be sensitive to the ethical dilemmas which arise in everyday life. For example, if twelve patients need their bed linen changing and there are only six clean sheets in the ward, a decision has to be made about which patients get those sheets. 'Ethical sensitivity' enables a nurse to see that this situation presents him or her with an ethical dilemma. 'Action related to a moral position' can be interpreted as the capacity of an individual to act in a way which she or he believes to be right for her or himself and for other people concerned. Such action, therefore, involves taking other people's views into account and being sensitive to the implications of one's actions for other people. Finally, 'commitment to a moral stance' can be interpreted as meaning that a person has reflected on her or his own actions and identified certain principles she or he will always stand by. For example, a person may be committed to the principle of never telling a 'noble lie'.

The author has elsewhere (Glen, 1988) used Rest's model to underpin the ethics component of a nursing curriculum (Fig. 2.3.). In order to discuss the moral education of student nurses, it seems helpful to identify and take apart components of morality in this way the better to discover the extent to which each component has a place in the moral

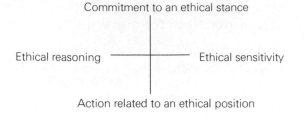

Fig. 2.3   Rest's (1983) Four-Component Model of Moral Development.

curriculum, bearing in mind that logical distinction does not imply psychological separateness, and that a dialectical synthesis will again be required if anything of use is to issue from this chapter.

Turning now to the work of Habermas (1978), it should be pointed out that his theoretical explorations into the nature of human knowledge and theory-practice relationships were not written within a context of educational theory, nor do they arise directly out of educational considerations. They do, however, have implications for the ethics component of the curriculum and for understanding associated pedagogical practices. Sarvimaki (1988) has also drawn upon Habermas' work to underline nursing's eclectic concerns. Habermas identifies three ways of knowing:

(i)   empirical analytic
(ii)   historical hermeneutic
(iii)   critical theory.

These correspond to what Harbermas terms three basic 'cognitive interests'; they constitute the three types of science by which knowledge is generated and organised in our society.

Rest's four-component model of moral development as it relates to Habermas' ways of knowing is diagrammatically represented in Fig. 2.4. The components of this integrated model will now be discussed further, with practical examples to suggest how the theory could be applied in practice. It should be emphasised that in the following discussion the learning activities linked to each component of the model are only loosely related in practice. For example, though the major thrust of a learning activity might be to facilitate the development of ethical reasoning, nevertheless other components of morality are likely to be involved also. In other words, the different components of morality cannot be neatly compartmentalised in practice as they can in theory.

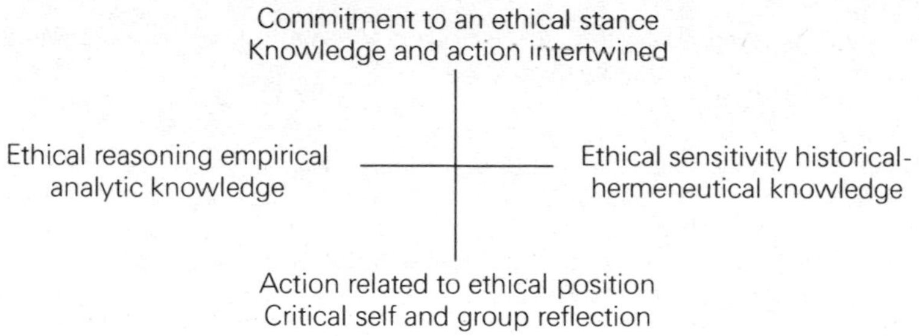

Commitment to an ethical stance
Knowledge and action intertwined

Ethical reasoning empirical ———————— Ethical sensitivity historical-
analytic knowledge hermeneutical knowledge

Action related to ethical position
Critical self and group reflection

Fig. 2.4 Rest's Four-Component Model of Moral Development as it Relates to Habermas' 'Ways of Knowing'.

Ethical reasoning: empirical analytic knowledge

Habermas (1978) identifies 'technical interest' as being congruent with the agenda of empirical-analytic science: [empirical-analytic science] 'comprises hypothetic-deductive connections of propositions which permit the deductions of lawlike hypotheses with empirical content'. This approach reflects a conception of a person as an autonomous entity which desires certain ends, calculates efficient means and acts in order to achieve the desired end. It is essentially an individualistic, highly cognitive concept. Empirical analytic knowledge is congruent with the cognitive developmental or rational approach to ethics, and, as Hide (1987) suggests, 'in this type of morality the knowledge base is a specific way of thinking in which the rules of logic or moral reasoning are "authoritative, consensual and fixed"'. Theorists such as Ehrat (1983) and Curtin and Flaherty (1982) have developed ethical decision-making models for the analysis of ethical situations in nursing, which incorporate the use of moral philosophy and principles. Others such as Langham (1977) and Mahon and Fowler (1979) recommend the use of Kohlberg's theory of moral development, suggesting the use of seminars for the presentation of situations which pose dilemmas, with the intention of providing the 'cognitive disequilibrium' in the individual student which Kohlberg considers necessary for progression to the higher stages of moral judgement.

The following learning activity devised by Beverley (1989), provides a worked example of a 'Kohlbergian' approach to the teaching of ethics. Students are presented with the scenario and in small groups discuss the ethical dilemma involved.

Emily

Emily Dickinson was a teacher until she retired at the age of 60 some 20 years ago. She has lived in the same bedsit in a large Victorian house in South Kensington for 30 years, comfortable in her spacious attic room on the 4th floor.

About 18 months ago, the resident landlord was alerted by several of Ms Dickinson's neighbours, that she was 'wandering half-dressed around the house' at all hours of the night, very confused, and unsteady on her feet. They also reported the fact of her double incontinence, and were continually having to clean up the common staircase and bathroom. In response, the landlord visited Ms Dickinson in her room, and found conditions of squalor; in addition, Ms Dickinson had no bedclothes, refusing the landlord's offer of some by stating that she did not need any 'in midsummer'. This was, in fact, January.

The landlord contacted a General Practitioner who visited, found her to be (a) malnutrite and (b) hypothermic, and arranged hospital admission. After two weeks' hospitalisation Ms Dickinson returned home. She refused offers of sheltered accommodation from social services (who visited daily), despite the fact that she remained very confused and incontinent.

Question for discussion: How would you resolve this situation?

This exercise was used with student nurses in the first term of their Common Foundation Programme at St. Mary's School of Nursing. The scenario provoked plenty of discussion, with different views being expressed about the dilemma. For example, some students categorically emphasised Emily's right to decide how she wanted to live, and got very angry with the landlord because of Emily's poor environment. Other students thought Emily should go into a home either because they thought she was a danger to herself, or out of consideration for the other residents in the house (Beverley, K. Personal communication).

Another approach is to identify key ethical concepts so as to facilitate a cognitive framework and promote integrated understanding in this area. Examples of this approach to curriculum design are Bergman (1976) and Seedhouse's (1988) proposed framework. The key concepts identified for this component of the Common Foundation Programme at St. Mary's School of Nursing include, amongst others, autonomy, justice, responsibility, authority and accountability (Bird, 1985).

Ethical sensitivity: historical hermeneutical knowledge

In contrast to the rational approach embedded in empirical analytic knowledge, historical hermeneutical knowledge is grounded in the fundamental need for us all to live in and as part of the world. It focuses on the need to acquire negotiation and communication skills. Hermeneutical knowledge is concerned with the refinement of judgement and understanding both of which are central to a caring profession. Philosophy has its limits. These limits and 'what in social and personal life counts as something' mean that a moral calculus, which underpins empirical analytical knowledge, will never displace the informed moral engagement and judgement of those in the caring professions.

Empirical analytic knowledge is associated with technical (instrumental) reasoning which involves calculating the most efficient means to achieve tangible results. Historical hermeneutical knowledge, on the other hand, is associated with practical reasoning which involves reflecting about means and ends together. Practical reasoning is discussed further in Chapter 10 in the context of curriculum decision-making. It is perhaps pertinent to note that within the context of the present neo-right climate of efficiency, effectiveness and enterprise, technical reasoning dominates in health care and public life in general (Elliott, 1988).

Hide (1987) notes that there is a large literature in nursing for this approach which is not seen by its proponents as moral education but as the teaching of communication and interpersonal skills. Authors such as La Monica (1979), Bridge and Macleod-Clark (1980), Clamp (1984) and Burnard (1985) recommend teaching techniques such as role play, experiential learning, critical incident analysis and the use of video tape trigger materials. This approach emphasises the social concept of a person, and as Langford (1979) argues:

'If the full social nature of the concept of a person is recognised there must be a corresponding recognition of the social nature of the concept of education. To be a person is to be a person living amongst and with others: it is to be a member of a community of persons ... he must learn to see himself and others as members of the same community, between whom understanding and with whom communciation is possible.'

(Langford, 1979)

Sockett (1988) has recently focused attention on some neglected virtues, including patience, conscientiousness, self-restraint and endurance. Many nurse teachers are reluctant to use such 'antique' terms as 'virtue' and 'vice' without apology, and this has led to a neglect of the disposition side of ethics education in nursing.

The following management exercise (Woodcock and Francis, 1982) has been used by K. Beverley as a values clarification exercise and it could help in the development of 'ethical sensitivity'. It is designed for use with groups of students who do not yet know each other or the nurse teacher. The fact that the exercise involves a fantasy situation provides a degree of psychological safety, yet it is an effective way of helping individual group members to begin to get in touch with their own values and decision-making processes. The students should work in small groups and they will require copies of the 'Cave Rescue Briefing Sheet' and the 'Volunteers' Personal Details Sheet' (see below). One member of each group should act as observer and should be invited to record the values being put forward, and the group processes. Recording the group processes, for example, would include noting how a view expressed by one student can influence the views put forward by other students. The 'Review Sheet' (see below) can be used both to give some guidelines to observers and also to provide an opportunity for observers to participate in clarifying their own values.

Cave rescue briefing sheet

Your group is asked to take the role of a research management committee who are funding projects into human behaviour in confined spaces.

You have been called to an emergency meeting as one of the experiments has gone badly wrong.

Six volunteers have been taken into a cave system in a remote part of the country, connected only by a radio link to the research hut by the cave entrance. It was intended that the volunteers would spend four days underground but they have been trapped by falling rocks and rising water.

The only rescue team available tell you that rescue will be extremely difficult and only one person can be brought out each hour with the equipment at their disposal. It is likely that the rapidly rising water will drown some of the volunteers before rescue can be effected.

The volunteers are aware of the dangers of their plight. They have contacted the research hut using the radio link and said that they are unwilling to take a decision as to the sequence by which they will be rescued. By the terms of the Research Project, the responsibility for making this decision now rests with your committee.

Life-saving equipment will arrive in fifty minutes at the cave entrance and you will need to advise the team of the order for rescue by completing the ranking sheet.

The only information you have available is drawn from the project files and is reproduced on the volunteers' personal details sheet. You may use any criteria you think fit to help you make a decision.

(Woodcock and Francis, 1982)

Volunteers' personal details sheet

Volunteer 1: Helen
Helen is 34 years old and is a housewife. She has four children aged between 7 months and 8 years. Her hobbies are ice skating and cooking. She lives in a pleasant house in Gloucester, and was born in England. Helen is known to have developed a covert romantic and sexual relationship with another volunteer (Owen).

Volunteer 2: Tozo
Tozo is 19 years old and a sociology student at Keele University. She is the daughter of wealthy Japanese parents who live in Tokyo. Her father is an industrialist who is also a national authority on traditional Japanese mime theatre. Tozo is unmarried but has several high-born suitors as she is outstandingly attractive. She has recently been the subject of a TV documentary on Japanese womanhood and flower arranging.

Volunteer 3: Jobe

Jobe is a man of 41 years and was born in Central Africa. He is a minister of religion whose life work has been devoted to the social and political evolution of African peoples. Jobe is a member of the communist party and has paid several visits to the USSR in recent years. He is married with eleven children whose ages range from 6 years to 19 years. His hobby is playing in a jazz band.

Volunteer 4: Owen

Owen is an unmarried man of 27 years. As a short-commission officer he spent part of his service in Northern Ireland where, as an undercover agent, he broke up an IRA cell and received a special commendation in despatches. Since returning to civilian life he has been unsettled and drinking has become a persistent problem. At present he is a Youth Adventure Leader, devoting much energy to helping young people and leading caving groups. His recreation is preparing and driving stock cars. He lives in Brecon, South Wales.

Volunteer 5: Paul

Paul is a man of 42 who has been divorced for six years. His ex-wife is now happily re-married. He was born in Scotland, but now lives in Richmond, Surrey. Paul works as a medical research scientist at the Hammersmith Hospital and he is recognised as a world authority on the treatment of rabies. He has recently developed a low-cost treatment which could be self-administered. Much of the research data is still in his working notebooks. Unfortunately, Paul has experienced some emotional difficulties in recent years and has twice been convicted of indecent exposure. The last occasion was 11 months ago. His hobbies are classical music, opera and sailing.

Volunteer 6: Edward

Edward is a man of 59 years who has lived and worked in Barnsley for most of his life. He is general manager of a factory producing rubber belts for machines. The factory employs 71 persons. He is prominent in local society, and is a Freemason and a Conservative councillor. He is married with two children who have their own families and have moved away from Barnsley. Edward has recently returned from Poland where he was personally responsible for promoting a contract to supply large numbers of industrial belts over a five-year period. This contract, if signed, would mean work for another 25 people. Edward's hobbies include collecting antique guns and he intends to write a book about Civil War Armaments on his retirement. He is also a strong cricket supporter.

(Woodcock and Francis, 1982)

Review sheet

1. What were the principal criteria used in ranking the volunteers?

2. How closely did the group's criteria line up with your own?

3. How comfortable did you feel about making this kind of decision?

4. What behaviours helped the group in arriving at a decision?

5. What behaviours hindered the group in arriving at a decision?

(Woodcock and Francis, 1982)

It will be noted in this exercise that the personal profiles of the volunteers are such that a range of values are likely to be expressed as groups try and reach a decision about the order of rescue. When the exercise was used with students in the first term of their Common Foundation Programme at St. Mary's School of Nursing, the participants were invited, in a plenary session, to give their perceptions of the values they had put forward during the exercise, and the group processes. After this, the observers gave their feedback to the whole group. Some of the principles which students tried to draw upon were 'Women and children first' and 'The younger a person is, the greater the right to life'. (The author is grateful to K. Beverley for these comments based on her experience of using the exercise.)

The next section focuses on a third component of the model in Fig. 2.4.

Action related to ethical position: critical self and group reflection

The distinctive features of nursing education, as adult education, might be seen as its capacity to enable 'perspective transformation' to take place (Mezirow, 1981). This rests on nurse teachers developing the students' capacity for critical reflection, for, paralleling Mezirow's notion of educating students for empowerment, Kemmis (1981) suggests that 'the sort of self-reflection within critical communities is emancipatory (because it emancipates) participants in the action ... from the dictates of compulsion of tradition, precedent, habit, coercion or self-deception.'

Moral educators using this approach do so through the examination of ethical dilemmas and debates from a case file of fundamental and topical ethical issues likely to confront a particular group or society long term. This approach therefore particularly facilitiates shared learning between professionals (Mackenzie, 1983; Watts, 1988; Brown, 1989). The plurality of opinion which emerges in the course of such a process of negotiation, conversation and inter/intra professional critical reflection facilitates not only a greater understanding of others, but also a greater self-understanding. As participants attempt to deepen their understanding, develop fresh perspectives and raise questions, they bring their own intuitions and unreflexively held opinions to focal awareness. Advocates of this approach include Thompson (1979); Boyd (1979); Campbell and Higgs (1982); Campbell (1984); and Thompson *et al.* (1983). Such reflective practice is potentially subversive (Lyneham, 1988) since reflection is a practice which expresses our aspirations to reconstitute social life by the way we participate in decision-making and social action (Labelle, 1986; Smith, 1989).

The following sessions, designed by Hawkett (1989) and based on her earlier work (Hawkett, 1988), could be used to facilitiate the kind of self and group reflection discussed above. The aims of the sessions are 'to enable students to explore the underlying philosophies which underpin nursing theory' and 'to promote a realisation of the importance of the students' own philosophy'. The sessions took place in the students' first term of their Common Foundation Programme at St. Mary's School of Nursing. The 60 students were divided into groups of 15, with two teachers facilitating each group. The following outline of the sessions is based on Hawkett's (1989) notes for facilitators.

Session One
Models in Nursing
(9.30–13.00 hours)

Stage One In this stage the theory underpinning the Diploma of Nursing in Higher Education was identified.

Stage Two Students were asked to 'consider and write down their own personal philosophies (what he/she as an individual considers to be the nature of person).' They were encouraged to draw upon the content of other course units to help them do this. The following list includes some of the aspects of the students' personal philosophies.

- Respect for persons – without this one cannot care for a person as a whole being.

- Each person has individuality.

- Individual people have worth.

- People are autonomous beings, their autonomy needs to be respected.

- All people are equal.

- People should not abuse their position and take advantage of others.

- Every life should be respected, not wasted, nor abused – this underlies the responsibility for how you use your own life.

- Selflessness is an ultimate part – but there is a need to respect and care for yourself, to have self-esteem if you are to be of any use to others.

- To be useful to others, one needs to be self-aware and very secure in oneself.

- Human beings are accountable to others and to God.

- Do unto others as you would like done to you.

- As members of a society we have a responsibility to look after other people.

Stage three   The students were then asked to consider in the light of their own philosophy, what they consider the rights and needs of clients to be. These were written down individually and then debated in the groups. Some examples of the students' views are given below.

- Patients have the right to negotiate decisions about care.

- To accept or refuse treatment, to respect, warmth and self-expression.

- To be treated as a person and not just as a disease.

- Respect for patients' intuition and insight.

- Right to nurses being available.

- Patients' responses and therefore needs are individual and must be respected, as such individual people respond differently and have different resources to draw on. Therefore you cannot expect, for example, that all patients will have achieved the same level of recovery a given number of days after the same operation.

- Right to be informed and to continuing education to stay healthy.

- Right to competent staff.

- Right to be listened to.

- Right to be an informed participant.

- Non-judgmental attitudes of nurses.

- To be treated as equal.

- Right to privacy, to be listened to, to be self-determining, to counselling and understanding, encouragement, equal care (no unpopular patients), right to availability of care.

- Right to be believed, e.g. 'Pain is what the patient says it is'.

- Recognition of what the person says; their needs, their pain, their emotions.

- Right not to be stereotyped.

- Respect for the person and their body, e.g. no bath if the person doesn't want one.

Stage four   The students were introduced to the Health Needs Curriculum Model which underpins their Diploma of Nursing in Higher Education course (Fig. 2.5). They were asked to identify the philosophy expressed in the model, i.e. 'what it says about the nature of the client and the nature of the nurse's response'.

Stage five Links were made between the philosophy embedded in the Health Needs Curriculum Model and the School's educational philosophy. The aim was to demonstrate that the values explicit in the Health Needs Model also operate within the Schools's educational philosophy.

Session Two
Building a Model of Nursing based on a
Personal Philosophy
(9.30–13.00 hours)

Stage one Students were asked to read the chapter, 'Models for Practice' in Wright (1986).

Stage two The notes gained from session one on the students' personal philosophies and their views about the rights and needs of clients were used as a basis for seeking to gain an agreed group philosophy.

Stage three The students were then helped to build their own model with the facilitators getting them to construct a framework which would enable the philosophy to be worked out in practice. (For example, this could have involved considering what knowledge and skills would be necessary to apply the group philosophy to client care.)

Stage four The students had now formulated a *global* philosophy/model and needed the skill of discernment to apply the model to different client groups. It was therefore suggested that facilitators should help the students to list what they considered to be the rights and needs of different client groups. The aim was to enable the students to distinguish between groups of clients and adapt the general philosophy/model accordingly.

Stage five It was suggested that facilitators should help students reflect on the process of the session, for example:

- It had enabled them to think critically, moving from an agreed philosophy to a theoretical framework which would enable care to be delivered in accordance with an agreed philosophy.

- They had done the exercise for themselves. They had not taken a recognised model and then tried to fit their own values into it. They had constructed the theory for themselves before being introduced to certain types of models. In the future they needed to be able to

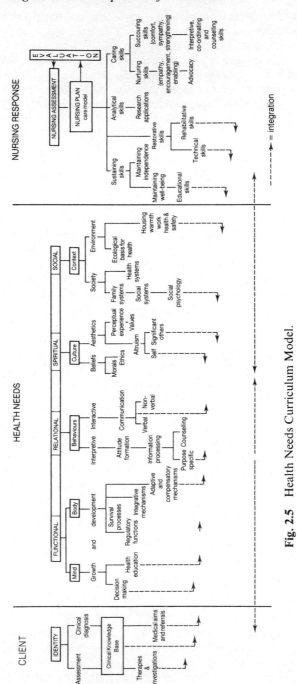

Fig. 2.5   Health Needs Curriculum Model.

ask questions about the appropriateness of various models encountered in different clinical settings.

The students found that writing their own philosophies was a difficult process because it required them to challenge their personal beliefs and affirm their values. However, the sessions were evaluated by the students as two of the best of the term (Hawkett, S. Personal communication).

These sessions are built upon throughout the Common Foundation Programme at St. Mary's School of Nursing. In order to facilitate critical thinking, to help students apply theory to practice and to allow practice to reshape and challenge theory, students are asked to observe the following during clinical placements:

- What beliefs and values operate here?

- Are they explicit or intuitive?

- What nursing approaches are used? Are they explicit, i.e. is there an expressed and owned model in use, or is the care intuitive and not expressed in a formal way which can be questioned and analysed?

- If a model is being used is it appropriate and is it working?

- What model best fits this client group and why?

Observations are kept in the student's Portfolio and are used in subsequent sessions on 'Reflection on Clinical Placements' and 'Models in Practice' (Hawkett, 1989).

Turning from an approach which stresses critical self and group reflection, the next section in this chapter will focus on the last component of the model shown in Fig. 2.4 (p.71).

Commitment to an ethical stance: knowledge and action intertwined

Commitment to an ethical stance is determined by a dialectical relationship between knowledge and action. Each component is required, and it is suggested that nurse teachers should work dialectically. In an article entitled 'The Reflective Practitioner in Nursing', Powell (1989) writes: 'With change in technology, social and environmental changes, and the advancement of nursing and social science research, it is important for ... nurses to be able to learn from their everyday work' (Powell, 1989).

This is equally applicable to the ethics component of the curriculum, and the following sequence is advocated by E. Pask (Personal communication). The student identifies an ethical dilemma from his or her own clinical experience, and is invited to discuss this with his or her tutor (Osborne and Martin, 1989). At St. Mary's School of Nursing the Common Foundation Programme students are asked to keep a journal in which they note ethical dilemmas they experience in their clinical placements (Aroskar, 1980). This helps the student to develop ethical sensitivity. The teacher introduces the student to any relevant moral theory and suggests the student analyses the dilemma in the light of moral theory. A written analysis might constitute a component of formative assessment process. This part of the sequence encourages the development of moral reasoning. The student returns to the clinical areas with, hopefully, heightened sensitivity and more coherent ethical reasoning ability. As he or she advances along the novice to expert (Benner, 1984) continuum, the 'Reflective Practitioner' develops a commitment to an ethical position which constantly submits to self and inter/intra professional critical reflection. It will be noted that the foregoing sequence relates to all the theoretical perspectives shown in Fig. 2.4 (p.71).

The following guidelines, formulated by Miller and Miller (1989), are given to the Common Foundation Programme students at St. Mary's School of Nursing, in order to help them with their journal keeping.

Cognitive–affective journals

As a part of the Diploma of Nursing in Higher Education course you are required to keep a Cognitive–Affective Journal. This is a journal in which you keep a record of your thoughts and feelings about your experience of being a student nurse (or any other experience you wish to include).

The recommended way to do this is to make a note of what you think and of how you feel about the experience. Having done this, make a Strengths/Needs list. This will serve as a record to help you see how you have progressed during your training.

It is hoped that you will feel able to discuss this with your tutor but it is important that you are frank with yourself. This journal is your property and is confidential. If you feel inhibited about discussing its contents it may be easier to copy part of it to discuss with your tutor. We would also encourage you to feel free to discuss aspects of your development with other tutors and clinical nurses with whom you have a good relationship.

The journal is part of the (formative) assessment process for the Diploma of Nursing in Higher Education and is a course requirement. The idea is that you learn to self-assess rather than rely on others for assessment. If it appears for whatever reason that you are not keeping a journal you will be asked to produce some evidence that you are.

Strengths/needs list

A strengths/needs list is a way of organising our thoughts and feelings when considering change and development or when evaluating our experience or arguments.

It is exactly what it says: on the one hand a list of the strengths of a situation or person, and on the other a list of the needs of that situation or person.

The strengths are those items which are positive, already exist and which are advantageous to the situation or person. The needs are those items which are not already present but which will enhance the situation or the position of the individual. The needs are positive items which will help.

The idea of the list is specifically to avoid the use of the word 'weaknesses'. Weaknesses are negative aspects which hinder. Identifying them may help decide the needs but there is little constructive use in identifying them for their own sake. Apart from the idea of a weakness being negative and restrictive it may not be relevant to the solution of the problem. It is far harder to accept advice if it identifies our weakness rather than points towards fulfilling a need.

Strengths/needs lists can be used for evaluating situations that we have been in, proposed situations, helping another person to make changes and for helping ourselves to make changes or evaluate the needs for change.

Formative assessment of the ethics component of the curriculum

It will be noted from the above that the journal forms part of the students' formative assessment and that it does not just relate to the ethics component of the Common Foundation Programme. This is because, at St. Mary's School of Nursing, the ethics component of the curriculum is assessed formatively as an integrated part of the Common Foundation Programme assessment scheme. The following information about the relevant written assessment is given to students:

Identify a situation from your own experience that had implications for client/clients' health needs. Analyse this situation drawing on sociological, moral, psychological, physiological and nursing theory. What were the implications for nursing practice?

It is suggested that the above be developed through formative feedback from personal tutor i.e.

1. Identification of situation by student — discussed with tutor. During this meeting student's own subjective interpretation of the situation may be explored and direction for literary search identified.

2. Formative feedback from tutor during development of essay. Opportunities for analysis and synthesis further identified.

3   Writing essay under controlled conditions.

Guidelines

1. Identification of suitable situation for analysis i.e. one that has implication for client/clients' health needs. This situation may have arisen in

any one area of practice i.e. hospital, community, mental handicap. It is anticipated that students identify clearly those implications for clients' health needs, that arise from the situation.

2. Evidence of analysis and synthesis which draws on relevant socio-logical, moral, psychological, physiological and nursing theory.

3. Implications for nursing practice clearly identified. Relevant issues con-sidered and discussed with reference to relevant research.

4. Full referencing and bibliography.

(Pask, 1989)

Conclusion

The preceding examples are intended to show how a dialectical approach to planning the ethics component of a curriculum could be put into practice. Notions like 'dialectical' are difficult. Our capacity for understanding them has been undermined by the vast success and academic prestige in recent history of scientific theorising and research. By looking to academics for the design of the curriculum, we typically find that they have formed something clear-cut and logical by declaring principles that should guide curricular design (Frey *et al.*, 1989).

Dialectical theorising does not go in for ready-made solutions or axiomatic forms of reasoning. The need to be open and invite debate and discussion between differing positions, if engaged in a spirit of communal search, offers scope and discussion between nurse teachers of different persuasions. Nursing education is too complex to allow us to back one kind of orthodoxy in the hope that it is a winner. Similarly curriculum planning and development must permit the co-existence of a variety of styles of reasoning, which stimulates dialogue between exponents of these various styles and ensures that intellectual pluralism in schools of nursing and health care in general is preserved and encour-aged.

The author is very grateful to the teaching staff at Parkside and Harrow College of Nursing and Midwifery for their help in preparing this chapter and Ursula Cowell, Principal, for her comments and per-mission to publish.

References

Apple, M.W.   (1979).   *Ideology and Curriculum*. Routledge and Kegan Paul, London.

Aroskar, M.A.   (1980).   Anatomy of an ethical dilemma: the theory and the practice. *American Journal of Nursing*, **80(4)**, 658–63.

Benner, P.   (1984).   *From Novice to Expert: Excellence and Power in Clinical Nursing Practice*. Addison-Wesley, Menlo Park, California.

Bergman, R.   (1976).   Evolving ethical concepts for nursing. *International Nursing Review*. **23(4)**, 116–17.

Beverley, K. (1989). Unpublished paper. St Mary's School of Nursing, London.

Bird, A.W. (1985). *Professionalism and Autonomy in Nursing*. M.A. dissertation. Institute of Education, University of London, London.

Bowers, L. (1989). The significance of primary nursing. *Journal of Advanced Nursing*, **14(1)**, 13–19.

Bowles, S. and Gintis, H. (1976). *Schooling in Capitalist America: Educational Reform and the Contradictions of Economic Life*. Routledge and Kegan Paul, London.

Boyd, K.M. (Ed.) (1979). *The Ethics of Resource Allocation in Health Care*. Edinburgh University Press, Edinburgh.

Bridge, W. and Macleod-Clark, J. (1980). *Communicating with Patients*. Joint Board of Clinical Nursing Studies, London.

Brown, C. (1989). *Perspectives of Staff and Students on 'Shared Learning' in Health Visiting and District Nursing Curriculum*. M.A. dissertation. Institute of Education, University of London, London.

Burnard, P. (1985). *Learning Human Skills: A Guide for Nurses*. Heinemann, London.

Burnard, P. (1988). Mentors: a supporting act. *Nursing Times and Nursing Mirror*, **84(46)**, 27–8.

Campbell, A.V. and Higgs, R. (1982). *In That Case: Medical Ethics in Everyday Practice*. Darton, Longman & Todd, London.

Campbell, A.V. (1984). *Moral Dilemmas in Medicine*. Third edition. Churchill Livingstone, Edinburgh.

Carr, W. and Kemmis, S. (1986). *Becoming Critical: Education, Knowledge and Action Research*. Falmer Press, Lewes.

Clamp, C.G.L. (1984). *Learning Through Incidents: Studies in the Development and Use of Critical Incidents in the Teaching of Attitudes in Nursing*. M. Phil. thesis. Institute of Education, University of London, London.

Clay, M. *et al.* (1983). Moral reasoning and the student nurse. *Journal of Advanced Nursing*, **8(4)**, 297–302.

Clinton, M.E. (1981). *Training Psychiatric Nurses: A Sociological Study of the Problem of Integrating Theory and Practice*. Ph.D. thesis. School of Economic and Social Studies, University of East Anglia, Norwich.

Crowley, M.A. (1989a). The entrepreneurial nurse consultant: a Marxist analysis. *Journal of Advanced Nursing*, **14(7)**, 582–6.

Crowley, M.A. (1989b). Feminist pedagogy: nurturing the ethical ideal. *Advances in Nursing Science*, **11(3)**, 53–61.

Curtin, L. and Flaherty, M.J. (1982). *Nursing Ethics: Theories and Pragmatics*. Robert J. Brady, Bowie, Maryland.

Davis, A.J. (1989). Clinical nurses' ethical decision making in situations of informed consent. *Advances in Nursing Science*, **11(3)**, 63–9.

Department of Health and Social Security Community Nursing Review (1986). *Neighbourhood Nursing: A Focus for Care*. HMSO, London. (Chairman: J. Cumberlege.)

Dykstra, C. (1981). *Vision and Character: A Christian Educator's Alternative to Kohlberg*. Paulist Press, New York.

Ehrat, K.S. (1983). A model for politically astute planning and decision making. *Nurse Educator*, **8(3)**, 16–21.

Elliott, J.   (1988).   *Education in the Shadow of the Education Reform Act: the Lawrence Stenhouse Memorial Lecture.* Centre for Applied Research in Education, University of East Anglia, Norwich.

English National Board for Nursing, Midwifery and Health Visiting   (1989).   *Project 2000 – 'A New Preparation for Practice': Guidelines and Criteria for Course Development and the Formation Of Collaborative Links Between Approved Training Institutions Within the National Health Service and Centres of Higher Education.* ENB, London.

Fenton, E. and Kohlberg, L.   (1976).   *Values in a Democracy.* Guidance Associates, New York.

Ferguson, K.E.   (1984).   *The Feminist Case Against Bureaucracy.* Temple University Press, Philadelphia.

Frey, K. *et al.*   (1989).   Do curriculum development models really influence the curriculum? *Journal of Curriculum Studies,* **21(6)**, 553–9.

Glen, S.   (1988).   *Nursing Moral Education for the 3Cs: Care, Concern and Connection.* M.A. dissertation. Institute of Education, University of London, London.

Glen, S.   (1989).   *Power for Nursing Education.* Department of Curriculum Studies, Institute of Education, University of London, London. (Unpublished paper.)

Habermas, J.   (1978).   *Knowledge and Human Interests.* Second edition. Heinemann, London.

Handy, C.   (1984).   *Taken for Granted? Looking at Schools as Organisations.* Longman, Harlow.

Hargreaves, D.   (1980).   A sociological critique of individualism in education. *British Journal of Educational Studies,* **28(3)**, 187–98.

Hawkett, S.   (1988).   *The Philosophy of Terminal Care: Towards a Common Philosophy and Curriculum.* M.Sc. thesis. University of Surrey, Guildford.

Hawkett, S.   (1989).   Unpublished paper. St Mary's School of Nursing, London.

Haydon, G. (Ed.)   (1987).   Introduction. In *Education and Values: the Richard Peters Lectures,* G. Haydon (Ed.), pp. 1–13. Institute of Education, University of London, London.

Hedin, B.A. and Donovan, J.   (1989).   A feminist perspective on nursing education. *Nurse Educator,* **14(4)**, 8–13.

Hide, E.   (1987).   Philosophical and ethical curriculum issues. In *The Curriculum in Nursing Education,* P. Allan and M. Jolley (Eds), pp. 35–55. Croom Helm, London.

Hide, S.E.   (1980).   *Teaching Ethics to Student Nurses.* M.A. (Educ.) thesis. Institute of Education, University of London, London.

Huxley, A.   (1932).   *Brave New World.* Penguin, Harmondsworth.

Kemmis, S.   (1981).   *Professional Development through Involvement in Action Research Projects.* Deakin University, Victoria, Australia.

Kohlberg, L. *et al.*   (1983).   *Moral Stages: a Current Formulation and a Response to Critics.* Karger, Basel.

Kohnke, M.F.   (1982).   *Advocacy, Risk and Reality.* Mosby, London.

Labelle, H.   (1986).   Nurses as a social force. *Journal of Advanced Nursing,* **11(3)**, 247–53.

La Monica, E.L.   (1979).   The nurse and the aging client: positive attitude formation. *Nurse Educator,* **4(6)**, 23–6.

Langford, G. (1979). Education is of the whole man. *Journal of Philosophy of Education*, **13**, 65–72.

Langham, P. (1977). Open forum: on teaching ethics to nurses. *Nursing Forum*, **16(3/4)**, 220–7.

Laurent, C. (1988). Mentors on hand to help. *Nursing Times and Nursing Mirror*, **84(46)**, 29–30.

Lovin, R.W. (1988). The school and the articulation of values. *American Journal of Education*, **96(2)**, 143–61.

Lyneham, J. (1988). The ethics of teaching ethics. *The Australian Journal of Advanced Nursing*, **5(4)**, 10–11.

Mackenzie, A. (1983). *Shared Learning: the Preparation of District Nurses and Other Health Professionals for Teamwork in Primary Health Care.* M.A. dissertation. Institute of Education, University of London, London.

Mahon, K.A. and Fowler, M.D. (1979). Moral development and clinical decision making. *Nursing Clinics of North America*, **14(1)**, 3–12.

Melia, K.M. (1981). *Student Nurses' Accounts of Their Work and Training: a Qualitative Analysis.* Ph.D. thesis. University of Edinburgh, Edinburgh.

Mezirow, J (1981). A critical theory of adult learning and education. *Adult Education* **32(1)**, 3–24.

Miller, R. and Miller M. (1989). Unpublished paper. St Mary's School of Nursing, London.

Morris, N. *et al.* (1988). Mentors: learning the ropes. *Nursing Times and Nursing Mirror*, **84(46)**, 24–7.

Myrick, F. (1988). Preceptorship: a viable alternative clinical teaching strategy. *Journal of Advanced Nursing*, **13(5)**, 588–91.

Osborne, L.W. and Martin, C.M. (1989). The importance of listening to medical students' experiences when teaching them medical ethics. *Journal of Medical Ethics*, **15(1)**, 35–8.

Palmer, A. (1987). *The Nature of the Mentor Relationship in Nursing Education.* B.Ed. thesis. Polytechnic of the South Bank, London.

Pask, E. (1989). Unpublished paper. St Mary's School of Nursing, London.

Piaget, J. (1932). *The Moral Judgement of the Child.* Routledge and Kegan Paul, London.

Powell, J. (1989). The reflective practitioner in nursing. *Journal of Advanced Nursing*, **14(10)**, 824–32.

Priestley, J. (1987). Comic role or cosmic vision? Religious education and the teaching of values. In *Personal, Social and Moral Education in a Changing World*, J. Thacker *et al.* (Eds), pp. 102–22. NFER-Nelson, Windsor.

Prophit, P. (1987). *Education for Productive Rule-Breaking.* Unpublished paper presented at St Bartholomew's Hospital School of Nursing's Annual Symposium.

Raths, L.E. *et al.* (1966). *Values and Teaching: Working with Values in the Classroom.* Merrill, Columbus, Ohio.

Rest, J.R. (1983). Morality, In *A Handbook of Child Psychology – Vol. 3: Cognitive Development*, J. Flavell and E. Markman (Eds), pp. 556–629. Wiley, New York.

St Mary's School of Nursing (1989). *Curriculum Document for Diploma of Nursing in Higher Education – Vol. 2.* St Mary's School of Nursing, London.

Sarvimaki, A.   (1988).   Nursing care as a moral, practical, communicative and creative activity. *Journal of Advanced Nursing*, **13(4)**, 462–67.

Schröck, R.A.   (1980).   A question of honesty in nursing practice. *Journal of Advanced Nursing*, **5(2)**, 135–48.

Seedhouse, D.   (1988).   *Ethics: The Ethics of Health*. Wiley, Chichester.

Shamian, J. and Inhaber, R.   (1985).   The concept and practice of preceptorship in contemporary nursing: a view of pertinent literature. *International Journal of Nursing Studies*, **22(2)**, 79–88.

Simon, B.   (1972).   *The Radical Tradition in Education in Britain*. Lawrence and Wishart, London.

Skilbeck, M.   (1984).   *School-Based Curriculum Development*. Harper and Row, London.

Smith, G.R.   (1989).   More power to you. *American Journal of Nursing*, **89(3)**, 357–8.

Sockett, H.   (1988).   Education and will: aspects of personal capability. *American Journal of Education*: **96(2)**, 195–214.

Spickerman, S.   (1988).   Enhancing the socialization process. *Nurse Educator*, **13(6)**, 10–14.

Thompson, I. (ed.)   (1979).   *Dilemmas of Dying: a Study in the Ethics of Terminal Care*. Edinburgh University Press, Edinburgh.

Thompson, I. *et al.*   (1983).   *Nursing Ethics*. Churchill Livingstone, Edinburgh.

Treacy, M.M.   (1987).   *'In the Pipeline': a Qualitative Study of General Nurse Training with Special Reference to the Nurse's Role in Health Education*. Ph.D. thesis. Institute of Education, University of London, London.

Tyler, R.W.   (1949).   *Basic Principles of Curriculum and Instruction*. University of Chicago Press, Chicago, Illinois.

United Kingdom Central Council for Nursing, Midwifery and Health Visiting   (1986).   *Project 2000: a New Preparation for Practice*. UKCC, London.

Walsh, P.D.   (1988).   Open and loaded uses of education and objectivism. *Journal of Philosophy of Education*, **22(1)**, 23–34.

Ward, K.   (1983).   Is autonomy an educational ideal? *Educational Analysis*, **5(1)**, 47–55.

Watts, M.H.   (1988).   *Shared Learning*. Scutari Press, Harrow.

Weinreich-Haste, H.   (1987).   Is moral education possible? A discussion of the relationship between curricular and psychological theory. In *Personal, Social and Moral Education in a Changing World*, J. Thacker *et al.* (Eds), pp. 54–64. NFER-Nelson, Windsor.

Williams, B.   (1987).   The primacy of dispositions. In *Education and Values*, G. Haydon (Ed.), pp. 56–65. Institute of Education, University of London, London.

Wilson, J.   (1969).   *Moral Education and the Curriculum: a Guide for Teachers and Research Workers*. Pergamon Press, Oxford.

Wilson-Barnett, J.   (1988).   Nursing values: exploring the clichés. *Journal of Advanced Nursing*, **13(6)**, 790–6.

Wilson-Barnett, J.   (1989).   Limited autonomy and partnership: professional relationships in health care. *Journal of Medical Ethics*, **15(1)**, 12–16.

Woodcock, M. and Francis, D.   (1982).   *Fifty Activities for Self-*

Development: A Companion Volume of the 'Unblocked Manager'. Gower, Aldershot.

Wright, S.G. (1986). *Building and Using a Model of Nursing*. Edward Arnold, London.

3 Using a nursing model in curriculum planning

Anne Casey

Nursing models have been with us for a long time. They are not a new or passing fashion. Nightingale and Bedford-Fenwick had strong views on the nature of nursing, the nature of the patient and the relationship between environment and health. The present concern with formal models is an attempt by the profession to move away from a medical and disease-orientated view of the patient towards an holistic and patient-centred approach.

The aim of this chapter is to demonstrate the influence of nursing models on nursing curricula. Following a discussion of the use of models, the educational implications will be addressed. The development of a curriculum for part 8 (Sick Children) of the professional register, using the Partnership Model of Paediatric Nursing (Casey, 1988), is presented to illustrate the place of models in the curriculum. This course was planned in 1987, hence it has been possible to evaluate the curriculum and, in particular, to confirm the views about models and curriculum planning expressed in this chapter.

Models of nursing

Nursing models can be described as 'formal presentations of some nurses' private images of nursing' (Fawcett, 1984). They are descriptions of practice providing a comprehensive and logical base for research, management and education. A model can be used to guide clinical practice by telling the nurse 'what to look at and how to interpret observations, how to plan interventions and how to begin evaluating' (Fawcett, 1984). The interventions which are planned and implemented should depend on tested theory. An example of the relationship between a model and tested theory would be that a model of paediatric nursing directs the nurse's attention to the child's inability to speak. Theories of child development indicate whether this is an abnormal finding and whether some form of intervention is needed.

The benefit of explicit formal models for practice is to ensure a unified approach to the patient. All nurses have their own informal models of nursing which guide the way they nurse. Confusion results if groups of nurses working together do not discuss and agree their team's approach (Pearson and Vaughan, 1986). Imagine the confusion for an elderly patient if the nurse on the early shift encourages him or her to care for him or herself, but the afternoon nurse does everything for him or her.

Models of nursing in the curriculum

In education, a nursing model clarifies what is meant by 'nursing' and describes what the learner is being prepared to do. If all nurse teachers impart their particular views of nursing the learners will be confused. This does not mean that only one model can exist. The use and development of multiple models are essential for the profession's growth and the prevention of a narrow perspective (Fawcett, 1984). This has led to an enthusiastic debate about whether a nursing curriculum should be based on a single model, or should incorporate many. There appear to be three options open to the curriculum planners (Pearson and Vaughan, 1986; Kershaw and Salvage, 1986; and others). One suggestion of these authors is that an eclectic model incorporating favoured aspects of several models could be the base for developing a course curriculum.

The second option is to divide the course into suitable modules or units and explore appropriate models in each unit. Flaskerud (1983) argues against this idea, suggesting that the students' knowledge 'can be expected to be compartmentalised with little carry over from one module to the next'.

Adopting a single model for developing the curriculum is the third choice and would avoid the confusion mentioned above. Other models would be explored as content within the curriculum, and their use in different settings discussed. The difficulty with this option for most nursing coures is that there seems to be no 'general' model which suits all nursing situations.

Most of the learning of nursing takes place in the clinical setting. This will still be the case when the educational changes proposed in Project 2000 are under way. So the single most important deciding factor in the 'models in the curriculum' debate is which models are practised in the areas where learners are placed for experience. If there is no established model, work is needed to develop clinical nurses' awareness of the importance of choosing an explicit model of care. Unfortunately models of nursing are being equated with time-consuming paperwork and 'academic' (i.e. 'not practical') care planning. With educational input, clinical staff can be encouraged to adopt, or develop, a model which reflects their view of nursing. They will resist the imposition of a model by educationalists which may require an adaptation of their current practice.

The process of choosing or building a nursing model has been well described (Aggleton and Chalmers, 1984; Fawcett, 1984). This is not a quick or straightforward task, but it is one which can be rewarding. Areas of good practice can be acknowledged and developed just by being brought out into the open. As nurses attempt to clarify their philosophy of practice and define the scope of their particular expertise, there is a new awareness of what they are aiming for and of what are the limits and proper concerns of nursing. Discussion of nursing models and theory can be stimulated and promoted by the continuing education of clinical staff and whenever changes in practice are proposed. At the Hospitals for Sick Children it was the Nursing Process Co-ordinator who was able to stimulate interest in models when changes were proposed to the nursing records. Because of her efforts nursing staff in the hospital were going through the process of adopting the Partnership Model at the time that the decision was made to plan a new course.

It was recognised by the curriculum planning team that a model of nursing was required to plan this new course leading to registration as a Sick Children's Nurse (RSCN). The decision to choose the Partnership Model of paediatric care was made for three reasons. First, it was felt that one model would be most appropriate for a 13 month course in a particular field of nursing. Second, the model seemed to describe practice in the areas where clinical experience was to be gained. Analysis and discussion of several existing models revealed, among other things, that there was insufficient emphasis on parental involvement and on the developmental needs of the child. Although the Partnership Model was new and relatively untested it was felt to be acceptable because of the positive responses of paediatric nurses in all specialties, including community care, when it was introduced to them. It did seem that a single model existed which could form the base of the RSCN curriculum.

The third factor was the consequence of choosing Lawton's (1983) Cultural Analysis model to develop the curriculum. The result of the cultural analysis (summarised below) was entirely consistent with the principles of the Partnership Model of care.

Before outlining the development of the RSCN curriculum, a summary of philosophy and key elements of the model is given to make this example more meaningful.

The Partnership Model of care

Over the last thirty years, radical changes have occurred in the provision of care for the sick child. It is hoped that, whenever possible, sick children are kept out of hospital, as recommended by the Platt committee (Department of Health and Social Security Central Health Services Council, 1959). In the past, provision of community support for carers coping at home has been inadequate, but the Griffiths report (1988) on community health care brought new hope that there would at last be resources to provide essential support and respite care.

If a child does need to be admitted to hospital, it is commonplace today for parents to participate in the care their child requires. 'Family-centred care' and care given in partnership with the family, form the basis of paediatric nursing philosophy for the nineties. The beliefs and values which underpin the Partnership Model include recognition of the family as the best people to care for the child. They are the experts in their child's care and the nurse must view each child in the context of his or her family, in order to provide the best possible care. In this model the *child* is defined as a unique individual who is functioning, growing and developing – physically, emotionally, intellectually, socially and spiritually. In order to survive and grow and develop children need care in the form of protection, sustenance, stimulation and love. Most of a child's needs are initially met by their family. The care that is given to help children meet their needs is termed *family care*. As children develop they learn to look after themselves, taking on more and more of their own care until they are independent and considered mature. A child's *family* is defined as the group which takes responsibility for helping the child meet his or her needs. They are not viewed as the 'patient'; a Health Visitor would perhaps define the family differently as they are her or his client group. From conception it is the family who mediate between the child and his or her environment.

A safe and suitable *environment* must be provided if the child is to flourish. Influences on the child's environment, which the family may or may not have some control over, can be cultural, social, psychological and physical. Children's surroundings not only affect their growth and development, but also their physical and mental *health*. The developing child who is healthy and well cared for will have the best opportunity to achieve his or her full potential.

In most cases of childhood illness the family are quite able to manage at home. However if they can no longer provide all the care that is needed, assistance will be sought from health carers. Nursing may be one of the forms of assistance required. The *paediatric nurse* complements parental care by doing things for the child or parent to meet the child's needs. This action may be family care, which is individual to each child and is the familiar, trusted routine that should be continued if at all possible. Or the action may be in the form of *nursing care* (that extra care which is required in relation to the health problem). For example; the child's bath is a home routine and is family care, until the child has an intravenous line inserted. Bathing the child with an infusion requires extra caution and some skill in removing clothing! This is the extra care which forms nursing care. Depending on their capabilities children may do some, or all, of this care themselves. To enable them to do this, and to assist parents who wish to be involved in all aspects of their child's care, the nurses's role is also that of teacher and supporter. The nurse demonstrates how to get the shirt over the intravenous site safely and stays with the parent until she or he feels confident to manage alone.

Working as a member of a multidisciplinary team, nurses recognise the limits of their expertise and refer the family to other team members when appropriate. Most nurses are not, for example, trained as counsellors. If assessment of a family's coping indicates that there are major problems, the nurse would consult with the team and refer to the most suitable member for expert help.

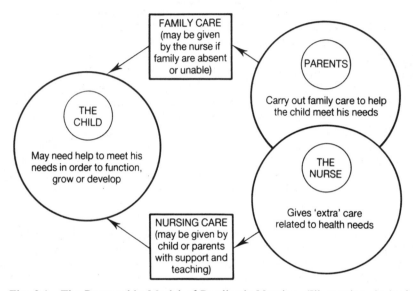

Fig. 3.1   The Partnership Model of Paediatric Nursing. (Illustration devised by K. Spires.)

The process of nursing is carried out in partnership with the family. Explanation of this approach allows the family to decide to what extent they would like to be involved in care. Part of the supportive care that is given by the nurse includes continuous re-assessment of the parents' ability to cope with this involvement, and the re-negotiation of care responsibility if necessary. When assessment indicates that a family do not wish, or are unable to participate, this is respected and the nurse tries to carry out family care as the family would do it. The diagrammatic summary of the Partnership Model of care (Fig. 3.1) illustrates the relationship between child, family and paediatric nurse.

Testing the model

Essential to the adoption or development of any model is to test it in a variety of settings and to make explicit the theoretical basis of the statements made within it. Many of the statements and assumptions included in the Partnership Model can be supported by existing research. Studies of children in hospital confirm the assumption that such children need their parents. The statements about paediatric nursing are mostly based on the beliefs of practising nurses, elicited in discussion and by questionnaire. The fact that the model is felt, by these nurses, to be an accurate description of their best practice helps in validating it. It is intended that the model is expressed in language that is understandable to parents as well as nurses.

A comprehensive study by Knafl *et al.* (1988) provides insight into the nature and effects of parental participation in care of the hospitalised child. There are lessons in this work for all paediatric nurses and many of the conclusions support the principles of the Partnership approach. Evidence from other unrelated projects (Webb *et al.*, 1985; Cleary *et al.*, 1986) confirm that parents are willing and able to perform many nursing tasks. However, a study by Gill (1987) emphasises that although nurses state that their care is family-centred, their attitudes to parental involvement may prevent full participation.

To be of use the Partnership Model should help develop practice by encouraging examination of important issues. At the same time, developments in practice and research into paediatric nursing will contribute to the growth of the model. By making this view of nursing explicit to peers and professional colleagues, it has been found that many issues which had been only vaguely addressed can now be examined in the light of a logical framework. Some of the most important issues have been in relation to the education of paediatric nurses. The huge changes in the delivery of paediatric nursing care had not been incorporated in curricula other than in a fragmented way. It was recognised that some unifying model was required in education, to help prepare the practitioners of the future.

Curriculum model

Whereas a nursing model provides a framework for planning and delivering care, a curriculum model assists in the planning and implementing of educational programmes. Lawton's (1983) cultural analysis model of the curriculum was felt by the planners to be particularly suitable for developing an RSCN course, at a time when nursing practice and education are being required to adapt to meet changing needs in society. This model assists the choice of content and teaching methods for a curriculum by providing a framework for identifying what are the valued parts of the culture which are to be passed on.

The starting point for planning a curriculum, according to Lawton, is to analyse the culture by considering the following questions:

'a)   what kind of society already exists?
b)   in what ways is it developing?
c)   how do its members appear to want it to develop?
d)   what kinds of values and principles will be involved in deciding on c)
       and the educational means of achieving c)?'

(Lawton, 1983)

Lawton's model was designed for general education but it is easily adapted to nursing if 'society' is limited to the groups immediately concerned. In paediatric nursing this would include the nurses, patients and families as well as professional and statutory bodies responsible for the regulation and development of nursing, and those concerned with the provision of health care for children. Analysis of the 'culture' of paediatric nursing 'society' should reveal all the factors to be considered in the planning of courses to prepare nurses to care for children. Lawton's four questions will therefore now be used as a means of analysing this 'culture'. (Information about the curriculum is taken from the Charles West School of Nursing (1987) Curriculum document for the post-registration RSCN course.)

The 'kind of society which already exists' consists of nursing practice and education orientated primarily towards the care of sick children in hospital. Both are traditionally based on a medical, disease-related model which is still evident in many areas. Although parents have generally been encouraged to stay with their children when they are admitted, the nature and extent of their involvement in care have not been formalised, nor have the implications been fully addressed.

Paediatric nurses have tended to be politically unaware and not adept at stating their views. This is particularly important at a time when traditional values are being challenged and resources are scarce. The status of paediatric nurses as a specially trained group is not irrefutably established – an important area for attention in view of the proposed changes to the education of nurses in Project 2000.

The 'ways in which the society (of paediatric nursing) is developing' reflect the view that children may need nursing at any point on the health/illness continuum and in any setting. The use of the Partnership Model in care is assisting in the extension of parental involvement, hopefully improving both parent and nurse satisfaction. The move away from physical, disease-related care to a more holistic approach is evident. Paediatric nurses are among the leaders in the nursing profession in considering the intellectual, social and emotional needs of patients and families alike. The introduction of pre-admission programmes, play and schooling facilities, patient and family education programmes and day case surgery are just a few examples of developments over recent years.

'Members of the society', that is the nurses themselves, appear to approve of moves towards community paediatric care. Distances and resource shortages are overcome in many areas by the setting up of paediatric community liaison and care teams, often with charity funding. There is awareness of the need to develop teaching and support skills to enable family participation. Furthermore, attempts to develop the research base of paediatric nursing practice are being encouraged at all levels. There is also an awareness of the difficulty of changing the attitudes of other professionals to the need for specialist training and resources.

The long term views of the statutory body are expressed in the outline for the Project 2000 Branch Programme in Nursing the Child (English National Board for Nursing, Midwifery and Health Visiting, 1989). This outline identifies the special knowledge and skills which that body feels are required to nurse the child of the future. Such a child will be a member of an increasingly pluralist society and his or her care will require nurses who are socially flexible and tolerant. Changes in the economy, in housing and social service provisions, affect the vulnerable members of society first. It is probable that new patterns of disease will emerge as environmental and social changes occur. Furthermore, continuing advances in medical treatment and technology, including information technology, require adaptability, especially the ability to transfer learning to new situations. The nurse working in any setting will need to be a problem solver and researcher.

It became clear from this part of the cultural analysis, that the Partnership Model was a major part of the culture which was valued by paediatric nurses at the Hospitals for Sick Children. The analysis also revealed professional, educational and other issues and constraints to be considered in the curriculum plan. These included the resources available, the requirements of the statutory body, recruitment patterns and the service requirements of the hospital. Such constraints were sometimes at odds with the educational philosophy of the teaching staff.

The 'values and principles' which were involved in deciding the educational means of achieving all this are those expressed in the educational philosophy of the School of Nursing. This philosophy was arrived at by discussion at school meetings over several months of draft proposals prepared by a small working group. The following is a summary of the final version of the school's statement of beliefs related to nursing education:

'Teaching staff at the Hospitals for Sick Children view learning as a lifelong process. New knowledge and skills are acquired through active participation in learning activities. Nurses undertaking post-registration courses are seen as adult learners with individual needs and abilities. Nurse teachers aim to facilitate learning by providing educational opportunities and by guiding students to enable them to achieve personal and professional goals.'

The close inter-relationship between the single model on which the curriculum is based, the educational philosophy, and the curriculum

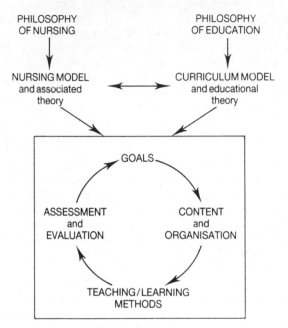

Fig. 3.2   Nursing and curriculum models.

model which helps to plan the course is illustrated in Fig. 3.2. The lower part of this diagram is a simplified version of the process which the planning team followed. Goals, or general aims, were derived from the curriculum and nursing models at the same time as a course plan, partially dictated by service constraints, was developed. Then the progression was as illustrated with other constraints, such as ENB requirements for assessment, being addressed at the appropriate time. The rest of this chapter will concentrate on the way in which the Partnership Model influenced the choice of the goals and content, the organisation of content, the teaching methods, assessment strategy and evaluation for the RSCN course curriculum.

RSCN course curriculum

Aims and content

All educational programmes must have a statement of intent. This provides direction for students, teachers and others, and serves as a basis for assessment and evaluation of the course. The broad aims of the

RSCN course were based on what the profession expects of paediatric nurses, drawn from the competencies listed in the Nurses, Midwives and Health Visitors Rules Approval Order, 1983 (Statutory Instrument, 1983). These aims included enabling students to develop the ability to help meet the physical, psychological, social and spiritual needs of children and families in their care. Students would develop the knowledge and skills necessary to assess, plan, implement and evaluate care 'in partnership with the family where possible, and recognising the inter-relationship of all aspects of a child's life'. Another aim was that the nurses would 'develop their ability to advise those who care for children on the promotion of health and the prevention of illness'.

The concepts defined in the Partnership Model indicated the breadth of knowledge required as content in the course. Essential to the nursing of children is an understanding of patterns of physical, psychological and social development. Considering the needs of the child for, for example, a safe environment, for food and drink, and to communicate, identifies content related to the maturation of the immune system, the gastrointestinal tract and to the development of language.

An understanding of relationships and normal stresses within families is important to the nurse who will be working with families at a time when anxiety about the sick child will increase stress. Economics and politics affect the family in a multitude of ways. In some areas of Britain the health of children is significantly affected by living conditions. The concept of Health is explored and the causes and effects of ill health make up a major thread in the curriculum. The cultural and ethnic background of the child and family may present difficulties for the nurse from a different background. Exploration of attitudes to others and increasing the nurse's knowledge about cultural and religious practices will help to bridge communication gaps between nurse and patient.

Associated with the concern for the welfare of all children are legal and ethical issues which affect the way children in different societies are treated. Environmental issues, health policies and resource implications form part of the course content so that the paediatric nurse can act effectively for the patients in her care.

Paediatric nursing is described in the model as a partnership with parents. In order to complement the physical and psychological care given by parents the nurse must learn parenting skills. Potty training and learning to feed oneself are not unimportant aspects of the toddler's life, they are not to be ignored in hospital and resumed at home. The key roles of the nurse as teacher and supporter dictate a significant part of the content of the RSCN course. Enabling the nurse to work with families begins in unit one of the course with communication skills and the theory and practice of teaching. Teamwork and group skills are included to promote the ability of the nurse to communicate on equal terms with colleagues.

Other nursing models for paediatric care are an important part of the content. It is probable that situations will arise where the Partnership Model is not appropriate. An older child who has been abused by a family member would probably prefer a self-care approach. Nurses must have knowledge of other views of nursing in order to be able to choose the most suitable model for their patients.

Organisation of content and learning experiences

Lawton (1983) suggests that curriculum content should be selected by analysing the culture according to cultural sub-systems which he has identified. Not all the sub-systems he mentions were felt to be appropriate to nursing. Those that were formed the basis of a further analysis, summarised in Fig. 3.3, confirming the content suggested by the nursing model. It also helped to organise the course by identifying some of the content threads which would assist in building up the students' knowledge and skills throughout the course.

Cultural system	*Application in paediatric nurse education*
Social and economic systems	Sociology (a) of the child and family (b) child rearing in a multi-cultural society
	Social aetiology of ill health
	Political issues related to paediatric nursing
	Experience in hospital and community with well and ill children
Communication system	Interpersonal skills
	Teaching skills
	Psychology
	Health Education
	Information technology
Rationality system	Research awareness
	Biological sciences (a) developmental physiology (b) infection control
	Nursing models and process
	Problem solving skills relating to nursing practice
Morality and belief systems	Ethical and legal aspects of caring for children
	Professional issues

Fig. 3.3   Cultural analysis applied; Charles West School of Nursing (1987).

But it was the nursing model which clearly indicated not only the essential threads, but also the emphasis to be placed on each of those threads. For example much more time is spent on the learning of teaching and support skills in this course than in previous courses. There is more emphasis on ethical issues, particularly related to accountability and parental involvement, and topics such as the sociology of the family are more prominent than in the past. All the threads are introduced in unit one and developed throughout the course as illustrated in the summary of the course plan (Fig. 3.4).

This plan of a course, based on a nursing model, is contrasted with planning using a medical/body systems approach where the nursing care lecture was always preceded by a doctor's lecture. The traditional curriculum was organised around the renal, cardiac, respiratory systems and so on, and was presented in the classroom as aetiology, investigations, diagnosis, treatment, complications, then nursing (Roberts, 1985). Substituting activities of living such as breathing, excreting and so on did not always alter the fundamental medical approach to patient care. In planning the RSCN curriculum to reflect a paediatric nursing model it became quite clear that the medical model was completely inappropriate.

In Fig. 3.4 content and learning experiences relate to the well/ill continuum (1) and to the type of care required (2). The dashed line indicates that the care may be given by the nurse or the family (including the child). Examples from the content threads for each unit indicate the way in which a progression was planned from simple to complex (3). Clinical placements (4) and learning experiences are closely tied to the curriculum content and teaching methods chosen.

Teaching and learning

From the statement of belief about the nature of learning, and from the cultural analysis, it became clear that the teaching and learning methods to be used in the RSCN course would be those which encourage independent study and learning through experience. In fact the curriculum planners opted to move towards a process oriented approach, reverting to the product or objectives model where specific products, such as clinical competencies, were required. Where appropriate, specific learning outcomes were stated, particularly for the learning of new psycho-motor skills. However students come to the course as Registered General Nurses, hence skills acquisition is not a large part of the course, as it might be for students new to nursing. Teachers and students are thus able to focus more on affective skills and on the development of the individual. It is only in this climate of flexibility that allowance can be made for students who come to the course with paediatric experience, who may be parents themselves, or who are more or less able.

WELL ←————→ ILL (1)

(2)

FAMILY CARE

NURSING CARE

PARTNERSHIP CARE

COURSE PLAN	UNIT ONE (the child in his normal environment)	UNIT TWO (the ill child)	UNIT THREE (the seriously ill child) (3)
EXAMPLE OF CONTENT	the rights of the child developmental psychology the family in society the child with special needs parenting skills common childhood illnesses	accountability in health care effects of illness and hospitalisation coping in stress and illness the abused child nursing skills caring for children following minor trauma	ethical issues related to intensive care sensory overload and deprivation helping others cope with stress the dying child advanced nursing skills caring for a child with an artificial airway
CLINICAL EXPERIENCE	COMMUNITY PLACEMENTS	LOW DEPENDENCY WARDS	HIGH DEPENDENCY WARDS (4)

Fig. 3.4 Summary of the RSCN curriculum plan; Charles West School of Nursing (1987). See text for further explanation.

Timetabling was to become more flexible with time allotted for self-directed learning. Some supernumerary clinical experience was agreed so that learners could practise skills, with supervision if necessary, but without the pressures of having to staff wards.

There is much research evidence about the way nurses learn to nurse which particularly emphasises the importance of credible role models (for example Orton, 1981; Ogier, 1982). The hidden curriculum which socialises novices into the ways of the profession can be more influential than any formal curriculum, especially when learners spend around eighty per cent of their course in clinical areas. There is little point equipping nurses with theoretical knowledge about the importance of considering a child's individual needs if, on the wards, babies are all bathed at 10 am and parents can stay but are not really welcome. When assessing the learning environment, consideration of the model of care practised is just as important as whether regular ward tutorials are held.

One of the principles of the Partnership Model is that the nurse respects the parent's expert knowledge. Nursing has been struggling for many years for professional status which, to some people, means jealously guarding their own expert knowledge. But nurses cannot work alongside parents without a two-way sharing of expertise. This is an idea that some nurses may find threatening yet what better way for a student to learn parenting skills than from an experienced parent? The hospital procedure for bathing a baby will be safe; but the experienced parent's way will be safe and will also be the way the baby is accustomed to having a bath. Teachers, post-registration learners and clinical staff may need support in exploring their attitudes and values to be able to step outside the bounds of rigid rules and procedures – a move which is essential if true individual and family-centred care is to be learnt.

A personal tutor system is one of the ways this support is offered to students to assist in the exploration of professional issues and personal attitudes. Clinical supervisors are an extension of the support available to students and these nurses play a part in the assessment of learning.

Implementing the curriculum

Before discussing assessment, it is worth spending a short time discussing the problem of introducing to learners, who may have completed a training organised on the more traditional lines, a curriculum based on a nursing model. The Royal College of Nursing (RCN) document discussing extended role (RCN, 1988) identifies the key issues, namely that medical tasks are seen as 'high status'. Medical knowledge is sometimes still perceived as more important than nursing knowledge. Intricate detail of disease pathology, for example, may be valued by post-registration learners above the theory and practice of communication skills.

Some learners will need extensive discussion about the nature of nursing, using an appropriate nursing model, before the relevance of some content is realised. Using the Partnership Model helps students begin adapting to the increased teaching/supporting role of the paediatric nurse, away from the 'doing-for' role they may have had in nursing adult patients. Of course a degree of medical knowledge is important in nursing. Relevant topics are included in content, but the emphasis has changed in courses planned around nursing models in that more time than in the past is devoted to the learning of *nursing*.

In a similar way, attitudes to teaching and learning may need to be addressed in any learners who have experienced more didactic methods in previous courses. These considerations apply equally to any nurse teachers who are accustomed to different methods and who may resist change. Curriculum innovation is addressed in Chapter 9 of this book and is of great concern to all who wish the success of new and important developments.

Assessment and evaluation

The assessment strategy for the RSCN course was concerned with discovering whether the students have achieved the aims of the course and whether they are competent to practise as paediatric nurses. The choice of both formative and summative assessment methods indicate the planners' commitment to assisting the individual to learn at his or her own pace, whilst ensuring the maintenance of standards. Difficulties in assessing communications skills were acknowledged but efforts were made to introduce self-assessment in as many areas as possible. This was seen to be essential for fostering the development of autonomous practitioners who would take responsibility for monitoring their own standards of care.

Continuous assessment of practice was introduced into this curriculum. The example given in Fig. 3.5 is taken from the documentation used in clinical areas during unit 2 (The Ill Child). All stages of the assessment reflect the nursing model in similar ways. The learners are encouraged to assess whether they have achieved these goals and confer with their supervisors to agree on the outcome. Areas needing improvement are discussed and future goals set so that progress is monitored, and the learner receives both praise for achievement and direction for future learning.

The most difficult task for the planners was the question of evaluating the curriculum. The work of Gallego (1983) was drawn from to make sure that all aspects of the course were evaluated. This meant that students' feelings and opinions were sought, as well as a consideration of pass rates and whether the aims of the course were achieved. Evaluation was continuous, repeatedly looking back to ensure that the curriculum was achieving all the developments in learners that were identified in the cultural analysis. One of the most difficult areas to

---

SECTION C: PLANNING CARE

Assess the student's ability to:

1. Plan how the child's home routines may be continued in hospital

2. Plan the care required in relation to the child's illness, investigations or treatment:

(a) physical
(b) emotional
(c) social
(d) intellectual
(e) spiritual

3. Negotiate with the family, their contribution to the child's care when this is possible

4. Participate in planning the teaching and guidance needed by the family to care for their child and assist his return to health

---

Fig. 3.5 Extract from documentation for continuous assessment of practice; Charles West School of Nursing (1987).

evaluate, perhaps because it had not been addressed adequately in planning, was the extent to which the nursing model was used in teaching. This reflects the need not only to prepare teachers for innovation but to evaluate the effectiveness of that preparation.

The curriculum used as an example in this chapter was developed and implemented in 1987. The process was a learning experience for all concerned and required many hours of patient work, particularly by the senior tutor responsible for curriculum development. This chapter may suggest that it was an orderly process: in reality it was fraught with difficulty and, as the end seemed to come in sight, the planners became aware that there is never an end. Internal evaluation of the course and the need to move towards Project 2000 have meant that many changes have been made. Development within the school of nursing have, among other things, increased the degree to which students can take responsibility for their own learning. New curricula for other courses incorporate the work of educational and nurse theorists more than is apparent in this example, particularly in the areas of assessment and evaluation. However the inclusion of the Partnership Model has been extended to all curricula and influences all aspects of those courses in the same way as described in this chapter.

Because this curriculum has been tried and evaluated it is possible to take a broader look at the way it was developed and to draw lessons for the future. With regard to the appropriateness of the curriculum planning model chosen, it is probably usually the case that in adapting any model, whether for nursing or education, favoured parts are included and others rejected. This changes the model and could leave it incomplete or give rise to inconsistencies. A less specific model than Lawton's could perhaps be wholly adopted for use in nursing education. Skilbeck's (1984) situational analysis model of the curriculum, whilst similar to Lawton's work, would allow the nurse educator to develop ideas about nursing and about education without being confined to cultural sub-systems that do not quite fit nursing.

The other lesson drawn from this overview is the importance of development and change. Society constantly changes and so must nursing and nursing education. As paediatric nursing knowledge develops, the Partnership Model of care will develop. It may well be replaced by other models more appropriate to the needs of the paediatric population. Likewise, revision and change in the curriculum will never end.

This chapter began with the statement that nursing models have been around for many years. As long as nurses continue to refine and express their particular approach to the care of others, models will remain an important tool in practice and in education. A model which defines nursing as an activity including teaching and supportive care will require the learning of skills appropriate to these activities in nursing courses. If the model defines a person as an individual with rights, who has physical, psychological and social needs, then ethics, psychology and sociology must be included along with physiology and anatomy. A nursing model, as an explicit statement about the nature and concerns of nursing, must be at the heart of all nursing curricula.

References

Aggleton, P. and Chalmers, H.   (1984).   Models and theories: defining the terms. *Nursing Times*, **80(36)**, 24–8.

Casey, A.   (1988).   A partnership with child and family. *Senior Nurse*, **8(4)**, 8–9.

Charles West School of Nursing   (1987).   *Curriculum document for the Post-registration RSCN course*. (Unpublished work.)

Cleary, J. *et al.*   (1986).   Parental involvement in the lives of children in hospital. *Archives of Disease in Childhood*, **61(8)**, 779–87.

Department of Health and Social Security Central Health Services Council   (1959).   *The Welfare of Children in Hospital: Report of the Committee*. HMSO, London. (Chairman: Sir Harry Platt.)

English National Board for Nursing, Midwifery and Health Visiting   (1989).   *Project 2000 – 'A New Preparation for Practice': Guidelines and Criteria for Course Development and the Formation of Collaborative Links Between Approved Training Institutions Within the National Health Service and Centres of Higher Education*. ENB, London.

Fawcett, J. (1984). *Analysis and Evaluation of Conceptual Models of Nursing*. F.A. Davis, Philadelphia, Pennsylvania.

Flaskerud, J.H. (1983). Utilizing a nursing conceptual model in basic level curriculum development. *Journal of Nursing Education*, **22(6)**, 224–7.

Gallego, A.P. (1983). *Evaluating the School*. Royal College of Nursing, London.

Gill, K.M. (1987). Parent participation with a family health focus: nurses' attitudes. *Pediatric Nursing*, **13(2)**, 94–6.

Griffiths, R. (1988). *Community Care: Agenda for Action. A Report to the Secretary of State for Social Services*. HMSO, London.

Kershaw, B. and Salvage, J. (Eds) (1986). *Models for Nursing*. Wiley, Chichester.

Knafl, K.A. *et al.* (1988). *Pediatric Hospitalization: Family and Nurse Perspectives*. Scott, Foresman & Co., Glenview, Illinois.

Lawton, D. (1983). *Curriculum Studies and Educational Planning*. Hodder & Stoughton, London.

Ogier, M.E. (1982). *An Ideal Sister*. Royal College of Nursing, London.

Orton, H.D. (1981). *Ward Learning Climate*. Royal College of Nursing, London.

Pearson, A. and Vaughan, B. (1986). *Nursing Models for Practice*. Heinemann Nursing, London.

Roberts, K.L. (1985). Conceptual framework and the nursing curriculum. *Journal of Advanced Nursing*, **10(5)**, 483–9.

Royal College of Nursing (1988). *Boundaries of Nursing: a Policy Statement*. RCN, London.

Skilbeck, M. (1984). *School-Based Curiculum Development*. Harper and Row, London.

Statutory Instrument (1983). *Nurses, Midwives and Health Visitors Rules Approval Order, 1983*. HMSO, London. (S.I. No.873.)

Webb, N. *et al.* (1985). Care by parents in hospital. *British Medical Journal*, **291(6489)**, 176–7.

4 Illuminating key concepts in nurse education: the contribution of sociology

Terry Maunder

This chapter discusses the contribution that sociology can make to nurse education, making reference to the five key concepts that the English National Board for Nursing, Midwifery and Health Visiting (ENB) (1989) suggest should form the major themes of the Common Foundation Programme of Project 2000 courses. Many of the ideas presented in the chapter stem from work the author did on planning and implementing the sociology component of a new Registered General Nurse Curriculum in 1986. The teaching of sociological aspects of nursing, using teaching methods that enhance student participation and teacher development, will also be discussed.

Rationale for including sociology in a nursing curriculum

Sociology is a social science: that is, it belongs to the range of disciplines (including history and economics) that concern themselves with the social behaviour of human beings. The author avoids giving a single, all-encompassing definition of sociology since sociologists themselves view the discipline from a variety of traditions and perspectives which establish that it is a complicated discipline. Sociology consists of a variety of ways of drawing conclusions about social phenomena: a Marxist analysis of these phenomena will differ from a Functionalist analysis, but each analysis will offer a unique body of knowledge to assist our understanding of the social world we engage in. Macro-sociological theories, such as the two mentioned above, examine societies and the implications of societal structures for the individuals living in them. By way of example, Marxist theories focus on the economic means of production, class systems and the divisions and conflict that these generate. Micro-sociological theories examine the effects of social settings, such as hospital wards, on subjective experience. One example of such a theory is Symbolic Interactionism which focuses on social relationships and the meanings people derive from their relationships through images, symbols, gestures and language. Such theories have constantly been reviewed, revised and elaborated upon as the discipline has developed.

The Registered Mental Nurse Syllabus (National Boards for England and Wales, 1982) acknowledged the importance of sociology for psychiatric nurses by including it as part of the knowledge base that psychiatric nurses require for effective intervention with patients. Since 'psychiatric nursing is a part of all nursing' (Doona, 1979) it follows that sociology has a relevance to all nurses providing care to meet the biopsychosocial needs of patients. If 'to educate means no less than to let someone exist, to stand out or transcend into existential space as the unique person he is' (Macquarrie, 1972), then the author believes sociological knowledge can contribute significantly to the development of nurses and nursing, especially since 'no consideration of an individual, whether sick or well, is of value unless he is seen in his social setting' (Chapman, 1977). Knowledge of sociology will develop nurses professionally and personally by providing a broader understanding of nursing itself, social relationships and a more sophisticated insight into patients' sociological and social needs. Peplau (1988) suggests that the quality of a nurse-patient relationship, and the therapeutic outcomes associated with it, depends very much on the type of nurse involved. If this nurse has the ability to integrate sociological insights into this relationship to help the patient understand him or herself or his or her world from another perspective, then the therapeutic outcome will have greater quality. This applies in any setting. Moreover, if 'the sociological imagination is becoming the major common denominator of our cultural life' (Mills, 1970), then sociology can be used for the development of nurses engaging in complex patterns of interaction.

Nursing models attempt to represent through core concepts (nursing, health, person, society) and empirical evidence what nursing is; they are 'developed logically, with care and effort, in an attempt to make better sense of what nurses do and should do' (Aggleton and Chalmers, 1984). They identify important components of nursing and the knowledge base and skills by which nursing intervention may be implemented through the tool of the nursing process. For example, Riehl's and Roy's (1980) nursing model borrows from the theory of symbolic interactionism to emphasise the way individuals interact through symbols, shared meanings, language and gestures. The nurse should enter the subjective world of the patient and see things as he or she does; for example, appreciating the stress that symbols such as technical equipment may generate in patients and assisting the patient to understand this stress and learn ways of coping with it. A sound grasp of such a theory applied to a model of nursing can provide even broader insights: an appreciation of how the word symbol 'Ward Sister' on an office door may influence the behaviour of people entering that office; an appreciation of how the symbol of a uniform colour and the status associated with it may influence the degree of trust a patient places in a nurse.

As a tool for the delivery of nursing care, the holistic nursing process requires that nurses engage in activities which most appropriately meet the individual biopsychosocial needs of patients; if part of the nurse's knowledge base is sociology then it follows that she or he will be better equipped to meet these needs and understand the activity called nursing. The profession can only be enriched by the nurse who can view the total delivery of care in terms of symbolic meanings, like those mentioned, as well as disease processes.

The following sections discuss the planning of the sociology component of a new Registered General Nurse curriculum.

Sociology in a nursing curriculum

The curriculum was developed through teachers working in task groups and the curriculum planning model was a modification (Studdy, 1985) of the Lawton (1983)/Skilbeck (1984) cultural/situational analysis models which take into account wider social and cultural considerations, thus enabling teachers to work toward a 'curriculum which sets out to orientate pupils towards the principal issues, trends and developments in contemporary culture' (Reynolds and Skilbeck, 1976). The curriculum planning model was selected for its congruence with the values and beliefs of the organisation and the ideology that education can be used for planned change. The Registered General Nurse curriculum (Studdy, 1987) commences with a Foundation Unit that is health-based before those units of learning that are based on the nursing care of the individual who is ill. The main themes of the curriculum are Nursing, Man, Health, Society, Personal and Social Development.

It was considered that there might be resistance to learning sociology on the part of student nurses. Barthes (1973) defines myth as 'a type of speech' that has become a system of communicated messages. These messages are not confined to oral speech but can be communicated through art, cinema, photographs, newspaper reports and other media which can support and reinforce oral myths. Since 'the universe is infinitely fertile in suggestion' (Barthes, 1973) and myth as a pattern of communication permeates our understanding of the social world, it is the case that the discipline we 'know' as sociology is clouded by myth. For example, the images of political activity by students are inextricably linked to the myth of sociology as the repository of class struggle and revolutionary ideology; the result of this is that 'students, however sullen looking and apparently self-obsessed, come to sociology because they believe it is concerned with people and that it contributes to the understanding and practical improvement of human relations' (O'Neill,

1972). Sociologists have much to contribute to our understanding of ourselves and the societies we live in, but they cannot read minds or presume to offer more to the public good than other social scientists. It should be borne in mind that 'sociology can be done in armchairs or buses, at sidewalk cafes or at university. Sociology belongs to familiar scenes, to neighbourhoods, gangs and slums. In everyday life, sociology belongs to the cunning of the salesman and the hustler, to the proverbial barman and taxi-driver' (O'Neill, 1972). To this end, it was intended that the sociology component of the curriculum would seek to develop nurses through sociological enquiry rather than producing sociologists who happen to be nurses; the priority was the development and delivery of well informed nursing interventions.

The goals of this component of the curriculum would not necessarily have observable outcomes, and some of the intellectual processes generated by some of the material presented were likely to continue after registration. In the achievement of aims and objectives teacher input would take the form of assisting learners to explore issues, enabling them to seek and formulate explanations, through experiences and discussion with the hope that the sociology component would also offer 'a high degree of personal and professional development' (Stenhouse, 1975) for teachers, while achieving learning outcomes for student nurses. It was anticipated that teacher-student encounters would allow for creativity of thought and expression.

As a proponent of discovery learning, Bruner argues that 'learning is so deeply ingrained in man that it is almost involuntary' (Bruner, 1966) and that the will to learn exists in all people. He maintains that a theory of instruction has four major features or criteria which may guide the activity of teaching: predisposition towards learning such as cultural factors; the structure of knowledge for optimal learning; effective sequencing of what is to be learned; and the reinforcement available to enhance learning. Discovery learning takes place when a class is organised so that the learners are actively involved with the result that learning becomes 'the kind of internal discovery that is probably of highest value' (Bruner, 1966). These features influenced the organisation of curriculum content and selection of teaching methodologies.

Where possible didactic exposition should be avoided since 'it is less effective for the promotion of thought and for changing attitudes' (Bligh, 1971); however, the nature of some of the content might not lend itself to totally student-centred methods. In such sessions an informal lecture style wherein 'students are encouraged to interrupt for questions, comments, and clarification' (de Tornyay and Thompson, 1987) should be adopted. Teaching methodology is congruent with teacher intention and proposed learning outcomes; 'progressive' methods are not selected for the sake of it or to meet teacher need. Consideration of teaching methods suggested that a variety could be employed, including experiential approaches like role-play, sculpting and games, to enhance the learning of knowledge-based topics. Debriefing and deroling procedures should be an integral part of such sessions. The following methods were also considered appropriate:

Method	Advantage
Brainstorming	Spontaneous suggestion and problem-solving.
Buzz groups	Quieter students can contribute, terminology is learned, arousal and group cohesion are increased.
Debates	Exploration of new ideas.
Projects	Active learning with improved presentation skills.

(Adapted from Bligh, 1971)

A basic reading list was provided, focusing on texts specific to sociology and nursing, for example Chapman (1977). It was expected that students would subsequently search out relevant materials themselves. Assessment of learning was by incorporating sociological aspects of care into the marking guidelines for theoretical assessments such as nursing care diaries. Students must demonstrate in written assessments that they have taken account of sociology as a discipline that has relevance to nursing.

The rationales, ideas, considerations and principles outlined above have a direct relevance for teachers considering the sociology component of Project 2000 courses, which will now be examined.

Possible sociology component of a Project 2000 course

The course development guidelines for 'Project 2000 – A New Preparation for Practice' issued by the ENB in January 1989 suggest possible content related to five key concepts that should form the major themes of the Common Foundation Programme and branch programmes. These themes are: *The Individual; Society; Health; Health Care* and *Nursing*. An examination of the aims of the Common Foundation Programme indicates that knowledge of sociology as part of nursing has relevance in relation to the provision of 'opportunities for students to develop their intellectual abilities, self-awareness and self-direction' (ENB, 1989) and the provision of experience for students that will 'enable them to communicate with sensitivity, observe with understanding, reflect with insight and participate in the delivery of care with knowledge and skill' (ENB, 1989). With regard to the suggested content in relation to the five key concepts, sociology has relevance in the following areas:

The Individual
For example:
   Exploration of self, self within a variety of roles and affiliations
   Presentation of self and self-awareness
   The individual as part of the collective

Society
For example:
   Socialisation and education
   Labelling and stigma
   Deviance as a socially constructed phenomenon

Health
For example:
   Reduced health potential as a consequence of social dis-
   advantage/deprivation
   Health determinants
   Definition of health

Health Care
For example:
   Health care structures
   Local, national and international policies

Nursing
For example:
   Definitions, theories and models of nursing
   Patterns of organisation in nursing
   Nursing culture

The above areas are examples and they are not exhaustive. An examination of the aims and suggested content of the branch programmes
also indicates the relevance of sociology to nurse education and the
preparation of new practitioners. For example, one aim of the Branch
Programme in Mental Health Nursing is to prepare practitioners to
'base mental health care within a framework which recognises issues of
race, ethnicity and gender as important factors associated with access
to service' (ENB, 1989), a process to which the teaching of sociology
could make a valuable contribution. Content statements with regard to
this branch also indicate that sociology should continue to be part
of the mental health nurse's knowledge base by recognising that the
Registered Mental Nurse Syllabus (National Boards for England and
Wales, 1982) continues to be relevant and suggesting content related
to, for example, 'multicultural dimensions', 'human relationships and
the helping process' and 'information utilisation'.
   The contribution that sociology could make to learning outcomes
would be in developing students' abilities to analyse social phenomena,
to explore the social world they engage in, to apply sociological insights
to nursing intervention, to seek sociological explanations of health and

illness and to understand self in relation to others and society. Such a process would make a significant contribution to developing students' analytical abilities and self-awareness skills while the teaching methods considered earlier will facilitate self-direction in learning.

Drawing on previous experience of planning and teaching sociological aspects of nursing, the author considers that the following content areas *might* be considered appropriate for part of a Common Foundation Programme. It is not intended to be an exhaustive content map.

1   Introduction to the Social Sciences
  (a)   The range of disciplines: psychology, economics, politics, for example
  (b)   Comparing social sciences to natural sciences
  (c)   The relevance of social sciences to nursing and health

2   Introduction to Sociology
  (a)   Sociological perspectives at macro and micro levels
  (b)   The relevance of sociology to nursing and health
  (c)   The focus of sociology enquiry: what do sociologists study?

3   Methods of Social Investigation
  (a)   The role and relevance of research in nursing and patterns of health
  (b)   Questionnaires, surveys and statistics in research
  (c)   Content analysis of historical documents
  (d)   Observation and participant observation

4   Sociological Theories
  (a)   Structural Functionalism – social systems, socialisation, norms and values
  (b)   Marxism – alienation, social relations, social deprivation
  (c)   Symbolic Interactionism – development of self, shared meanings, symbols in society
  (d)   The relationship between sociological theory, nursing and health

5   Urban Sociology: The Community
  (a)   The urban milieu: Durkheim – mechanical versus organic solidarity; Tönnies – Community versus Association
  (b)   Urban deprivation and health

6   Sociological Aspects of Patient Population
  (a)   The relationship between health and age, sex/marital status, religion, race/nationality, occupation/income, education, social deprivation

(b) Sickness behaviour – difficulties in definitions of illness and health: sociological explanations; factors affecting action when health status is threatened; differential use of health services according to class, sex, age

(c) Becoming a patient – the sick role, labelling, stigma, deviance; the nature of hospital care, for example, institutionalisation and its effect on health; the sociology of institutions, the total institution

7 *Family Health*

(a) Sociology of the family – extended, nuclear and symmetrical

(b) The family as a social system – roles in the family, conflict and health

8 *Social Structure and Health*

(a) Theories of social structure – Pluralism, Élites and Ruling Class

(b) Social order and social change – inequality/class and health

9 *Sociology of Education*

(a) The function of education – power, authority, socialisation, educational opportunity and class, social mobility

(b) Education and health – differential use of health services.

Readers will be able to assess for themselves which of the five major themes the above potential content relates to; the above examples should serve to demonstrate the very positive and meaningful contribution that the teaching of sociology could make to the professional and personal development of student nurses on a Common Foundation Programme. That said, the following presents ways in which sociological concepts and issues can be taught (and related to the five major themes) using an interactive approach to teaching and learning.

Teaching sociology to nurses

Experiential learning occurs when learners engage in an activity, reflect upon the activity, draw insights from the experience and subsequently internalise these insights into their behaviour. Experiential techniques enable learners to examine their feelings, attitudes and behaviour and also those of their peers. These techniques have evolved from student-centred philosophies of education and humanistic psychology which take the point of view that all human beings are motivated to grow and learn and 'have the urge to expand, extend, become autonomous, develop and mature' (Rogers, 1961). Experiential learning is usually associated with techniques such as role play, sculpting and games, although lectures also have the potential to contain an experiential component if a learner gains personal meaning from them; for example, a recently bereaved learner attending a lecture on the grieving process may gain insight into his or her feelings and behaviour. There are, in the author's view, certain *procedural principles* which should be observed when adopting an experiential approach to teaching and learning.

1 Where possible, (and sometimes this is essential), two teachers should be present: one to lead and facilitate, the other to monitor student reactions and teacher responses leading to ...

2 The principle of co-supervision following experiential sessions. Co-supervision is a reconstruction of the lesson, identifying strengths and weaknesses of teacher input and modifications for future sessions.

3 Teachers using such techniques should never expose students to experiences they are not also prepared to expose themselves to.

4 Teachers should be adequately prepared for using such techniques. If not experienced in their use it is advisable to seek supervision, and to begin with 'simple' exercises.

5 These techniques can produce strong feelings in both students and teachers (hence co-supervision) and teachers should consider before-hand how to facilitate unexpected reactions: one question teachers might ask is 'What is the worst thing that could happen in this session and what are my options if it does?' Practice runs with other teachers are useful for peer feedback.

The following provides an account of some sessions involving the use of experiential techniques in the teaching of sociology.

Introduction to Sociology: key concept – society

This can be facilitated as a three hour workshop using a peer group teaching approach. The following guidelines are circulated four or five weeks prior to the workshop.

Guidelines for Sociology Workshop
'I noticed that whenever learning involved either (1) creativity from the individual (2) personal choice by the student in determining a project or (3) controversy around an issue applicable to their personal world; learning invariably occurred, lasted and something intangible flourished for us all.'
G. Swenson (1974) quoted in Rogers, C. (1983). Freedom to Learn for the 80's. Charles Merrill, Columbus, Ohio.
1.   Divide yourselves into three groups.
2.   Each group has one hour to present a major sociological theory to the rest of the group:
Group one Structural Functionalism
Group two Marxism
Group three Symbolic Interactionism
3.   You will find sociological texts in section 34 of the Library.

4.   Present the key components of the theory and its relevance to nursing and health.
5.   Be as creative and original as you can; you can use music, literature, art to illustrate or reinforce issues. There are no constraints!!
6.   Teachers from your tutorial team will be present, but it is the responsibility of each group to ensure that the group ground rules are observed.
7.   The audio-visual technicians are on the third floor if you need them. My office is on the 11th floor.

T.M. 1987

In facilitating this workshop the guidelines have been found to be adequate for students to maximise their creative potential, and the workshops thus far have indicated that sociology, if introduced in this way, can be taught in a lively, student-centred way that stimulates interest in the subject. Effective use has been made of audio-visual aids such as overhead projector transparencies and handouts to convey information. Questioning by, and discussion with, peers have indicated that self-directed exploration of the theories enhance the likelihood of students beginning to *think sociologically* about issues and their relevance to their world of nursing. Students have devised and simulated scenarios (in relation to Marxism) which depict life situations that are alienating, for example, working on the production line in a factory; have written songs to depict the main components of a theory, for example, a song called 'The Symbolic Interaction' based on 'The Locomotion' by Little Eva ('Everybody's doing the symbolic interaction ...'); have devised exercises that explore the shared interpretations of non-verbal communication by asking the rest of the group what certain gestures and mannerisms mean; have devised scenarios which depict the different roles individuals adopt in social situations, for example, going to see your doctor. Music and literature have been used creatively and appropriately on some occasions.

The author facilitated these workshops in a non-directive fashion, acting as an educational consultant to clarify issues. For teachers attending the workshop the important thing to remember is that the students have prime responsibility for what happens in the classrooms and that they, the teachers, should relinquish control. Written evaluation has suggested that students both benefit from, and enjoy, this workshop, not least because it gives them an opportunity to work together.

A workshop approach could have wide applicability in the teaching of sociology, beyond the introductory level described. In terms of teacher development, this approach is useful in learning the skills of giving students total responsibility and resisting the urge to re-establish control if students reach an impasse in discussion, thus giving them permission to grapple with ideas or issues and find their own answers.

The Sociology of deviance: key concept – society

This session – which is *always* held with a co-facilitator – uses exercises modified from 'The Ingroup' in Pfeiffer, J. and Jones, J. (1974). *A Handbook of Structured Exercises*. University Associates, La Jolla, California, and 'Air-Raid Shelter' in Brandes, D. and Phillips, H. (1979). *The Gamesters Handbook*. Hutchinson, London.

Procedure

1.   Divide the group into small groups of 5–6 people.
2.   Each small group will devise a list of consensually agreed criteria by which one member will be excluded. Allow 20 to 25 minutes. Teachers should be alert to sabotage behaviour; each group *must* exclude one member.
3.   Each excluded member of small groups form their own group in a corner of the classroom and are blindfolded (optional). The non-excluded members form a large group again. They are instructed *not* to communicate with the excluded group in any way.
4.   The (non-excluded) large group play 'Air-Raid Shelter' with the variation that they also build a shelter with the materials in the classroom. The lead facilitator promotes discussion, following the exercise, on role stereotypes, power, alliance and scape-goating in groups. The second facilitator discreetly monitors behaviour in the excluded group.
5.   The excluded group are brought back into the large group in a 'goldfish bowl' by the second facilitator and asked to identify the criteria by which they were excluded, what it was like being excluded and how they feel toward those who excluded them. Teachers should be alert in this discussion to potential denial of true feelings, for example students saying, in an angry tone of voice, that they feel no antagonism to those who excluded them. Teachers should decide beforehand how this should be handled.
6.   The small groups reconvene and welcome the excluded individuals back both verbally and non-verbally. Each member then takes it in turn to state who they are, what they are doing and one thing they are looking forward to doing that evening (deroling procedure).
7.   After confirming that deroling has occurred, the teachers link the experience of excluding/being excluded to the processes of primary and secondary deviance, deviancy amplification and stigmatisation. This can be done by open-ended questioning to elicit the meaning of the exercise from the group or via handout and discussion.

As a means of teaching deviance and stigma this 2–3 hour session has a very powerful impact – only teachers confident in their ability to use experiential techniques should adopt this approach. The excluded group usually adopt deviant forms of behaviour in order to sabotage 'Air-Raid Shelter' and may go as far as leaving the classroom. Teachers should prepare for such eventualities and should remain on after the session to provide an opportunity for individual students to process any 'unfinished business'. It is not recommended that teachers go straight from this session to another one because of the potential feelings that might be evoked by exposing students to a negative experience of this sort. For the same reason, there *must* be two teachers in the classroom for this session.

Labelling theory: key concept – society

In this session, the author uses a modification of 'Headbands' from Pfeiffer, J. and Jones, J. (1974) ibid. to explore labelling and its impact on people.

Procedure

1. Invite seven participants to sit in the centre of the group. They are not to communicate with each other or the outside group. The latter should not communicate with the group in the centre.

2. Attach the 'headbands' on the foreheads of the centre group in a way that the person being labelled cannot see what the label says. The following labels could be used:

    Stupid – Ignore me
    Fool – Laugh at me
    Stirrer – Tell me off
    Scapegoat – Blame me
    Liar – Don't believe me
    Boss – Obey me
    Loser – Pity me

3. They and the rest of the group read the labels *without comment*.

4. The 'players' are given a situation to discuss: for example, a party in the nurses' home that got out of hand. The party was organised by the centre group and they have to give an account of it to the home warden. They are instructed to respond only to the labels of the other 'players', without using, for example, the word 'Fool' but demonstrating the behaviour, that is, 'laugh at me'. They are given a few moments to consider how to respond to each given label.

5. The 'players' discuss the situation for 7–10 minutes. Following the exercise, the 'players' are asked (still wearing their labels, without communicating with anybody) to write down:

(a) What does your label say?
(b) How did the others behave towards you?
(c) How did you *feel* during the discussion?

The observers, in groups of 4–5, are asked to write down:

(a) What happened?
(b) How can you relate what happened to your previous personal experience?
(c) How can you relate what happened to nursing and health issues?

6. Each 'player' shares his or her conclusions, as does a spokesperson from each group of observers.

7. The 'players' are invited to remove their labels and derole.

Opportunity is made for them to add any verbal comments they may wish to make about the exercise. This is followed by a discussion on labelling theory and self-fulfilling prophecies.

Variation
Depending on group trust and cohesiveness, individuals can be asked to identify their own personal labels or the label(s) of the group. Where did these labels come from?

While there is usually an element of humour to this exercise, it nevertheless has a powerful impact. Teachers should be alert to not giving a 'player' a label that actually describes that person. In some instances, it may be necessary for the facilitator and co-facilitator to use more than one deroling exercise; this necessitates teachers having a broad repertoire of deroling procedures. Students usually guess their label quite accurately and it is important to ensure that they leave the label behind in the classroom.

Family health and family dynamics: key concept – the individual

The following exercise is used to explore health-related aspects of family life such as roles adopted by members, family norms and values, power and conflict in relationships and patterns of communication between members. The exercise involves role play and sculpting and takes 2–3 hours.

Procedure
1. Obtain 'family' from members of group suggesting who should represent it, for example, mother, father, son, daughter, son-in-law, grandmother.
2. Ask for volunteers to role play this family.
3. Ask for 'presenters' who brief each volunteer on how to play their role. This is done separately from the rest of the group. 'Presenters' may, for example, wish the 'father' to take a passive role in the family, 'son' to take charge, 'son-in-law' to opt out.
4. While this is happening, the teacher instructs the rest of the group to act as observers or sculptors.
5. Observers are to identify the following during the role play:
(a) Conflict between members.
(b) Roles – nourisher, opter out, for example.
(c) Alliances and supportive relationships.
(d) Power – who influences whom, when, how.
(e) Communication patterns.

(f) Rules, norms and values.

They also draw a sociogram of interaction between the 'family'.

6. Sculptors are given examples of how sculpting can be used to demonstrate relationships. They are given time to practise. Two teachers in the session means (5) and (6) can be done simultaneously.

7. The 'family' act out the chosen situation, for example, 'Sunday lunchtime'. They have 20 minutes to do this; at which point the teacher draws a halt to proceedings.

8. Still in role, each member is asked what feelings and thoughts they experienced during the situation.

9. Sculptors then sculpt the 'family' to represent relationships, for example, a passive 'father' may be sculpted crouched on the floor under the 'dining table'. They then sculpt the 'family' to represent preferred relationships, for example, 'father' sitting at the 'dining' table with an assertive posture. For each 'family' sculpt, ask the members how it felt to be manoeuvred into these positions.

10. Invite observers to say what they saw. Ensure that the 'family' are referred to by role ('mother', 'son-in-law') and not personal name.

11. Individual sociograms (drawn during the role play) are displayed. The 'family' are then deroled.

12. The teacher then facilitates a discussion based around such issues as:

(a) How healthy was that family?
(b) What would happen to a member of that family who became ill?
(c) How might family dynamics contribute to ill-health?
(d) What should nurses bear in mind when nursing patients in the community?
(e) How far should families participate in the nursing care of a patient? What criteria would they use to involve/prevent family participation in that nursing care? Are there ethical considerations?

This exercise works effectively as a means of exploring sociological aspects of the family. It has been found that the 'family' situation presented for role play is usually negative and/or destructive. Teachers should therefore be alert to the fact that members of the student group may belong to such families and that the role play/sculpting may evoke personally unpleasant memories. It is advisable to stay behind in the classroom after the session so that any individual student who experiences this can talk to the teacher about it, if they so choose.

The types of session indicated here can be evaluated by the 'closing round' technique, which involves asking each learner to complete an unfinished sentence in the way they choose. Examples of such 'closing rounds' are:

(a) What I liked least/most about that session was ...
(b) One thing I discovered in that session was ...

(c)   One insight I'm taking from this session is ...
Other options include asking students to make a verbal pledge about
their future behaviour in relation to the issue (for example, exclusion)
or writing an open letter to the teachers about the session.

Co-supervision can be fruitful for evaluating and exploring such
strategies for teaching sociology. It provides an opportunity to analyse
teaching interventions and identify alternatives. In this sense, it is an
experiential process in itself and should be seen as a necessity rather
than a luxury. Student evaluations indicate that using experiential
techniques for teaching sociology is effective, even though some of the
exercises can evoke discomfort. It is important to create a climate of
trust so that such feelings can be expressed openly and without judgement. When meeting groups for the first time it may be useful to make
clear the rationale for the use of such techniques, emphasising that they
are based on educational theory. There are a wide range of texts
available, containing exercises that can be used as indicated in the text
or modified to suit individual taste or skill.

Sociology is an important component of nursing, both in terms of
knowledge base and nursing skills. The teaching of sociology facilitates
an understanding of both self and society; both are vital to good quality
nursing practice. Sociology can be used to teach content related to the
aims and five key concepts of the Common Foundation Programme of
Project 2000; The Individual; Society; Health; Health Care and Nursing
(ENB, 1989). Sociology can be taught meaningfully using student-
centred, interactive techniques which, through co-supervision, also
facilitate teacher development in the use of such techniques. Examination of the aims and suggested content of the branch programmes
of Project 2000 also indicate that sociology has a key part to play in
helping nurses develop specialist skills and knowledge. By continuing
to incorporate sociology into nursing curricula potential and current
practitioners will be able more effectively to integrate theory and practice to meet the holistic needs of patients. The processes described
have been demanding and exciting. Sociology, despite the myths that
surround it, has something to offer us all, whether in classroom or taxi!

References

Aggleton, P. and Chalmers, H.   (1984).   Models and theories: defining the
    terms. *Nursing Times*, **80(36)**, 24–8.
Barthes, R.   (1973).   *Mythologies*. Paladin, London.
Bligh, D.A.   (1971).   *What's the Use of Lectures?* Bligh, Exeter.
Bruner, J.   (1966).   *Toward a Theory of Instruction*. Belknap Press for
    Harvard University Press, Cambridge, Massachusetts.
Chapman, C.M.   (1977).   *Sociology for Nurses*. Bailliere Tindall, London.

de Tornyay, R. and Thompson, M.A.   (1987).   *Strategies for Teaching Nursing.* Third edition. Wiley, New York.

Doona, M.E.   (1979).   *Travelbee's Intervention in Psychiatric Nursing.* Second edition. F.A. Davis, Philadelphia, Pennysylvania.

English National Board for Nursing, Midwifery and Health Visiting   (1989).   *Project 2000 – 'A New Preparation for Practice': Guidelines and Criteria for Course Development and the Formation of Collaborative Links Between Approved Training Institutions Within the National Health Service and Centres of Higher Education.* ENB, London.

Lawton, D.   (1983).   *Curriculum Studies and Educational Planning.* Hodder & Stoughton, London.

Macquarrie, J.   (1972).   *Existentialism.* World Publishing Company, New York.

Mills, C.W.   (1970).   *The Sociological Imagination.* Pelican, Harmondsworth.

National Boards for England and Wales   (1982).   *Syllabus of Training 1982: Professional Register – Part 3 (Registered Mental Nurse).* ENB, London.

O'Neill, J.   (1972)   *Sociology as a Skin Trade.* Heinemann, London.

Peplau, H.E.   (1988).   *Interpersonal Relations in Nursing.* Macmillan, Basingstoke.

Reynolds, J. and Skilbeck, M.   (1976).   *Culture and the Classroom.* Open Books, London.

Riehl, J.P. and Roy, C.   (1980).   *Conceptual Models for Nursing Practice.* Second edition. Appleton-Century-Crofts, New York.

Rogers, C.   (1961).   *On Becoming a Person.* Constable, London.

Skilbeck, M.   (1984).   *School-Based Curriculum Development.* Harper and Row, London.

Stenhouse, L.   (1975).   *An Introduction to Curriculum Research and Development.* Heinemann, London.

Studdy, S.J.   (1985).   *Working Paper.* St Bartholomew's College of Nursing and Midwifery, London. (Unpublished).

Studdy, S.J.   (1987).   *Registered General Nurse Curriculum Submission Document.* St Bartholomew's College of Nursing and Midwifery, London. (Unpublished.)

5 Student-centred learning: facing the challenge

Jacqueline Bryan

'We assume that one of the main aims of education should be that of encouraging autonomous learning, and that consequently the relationship between teacher and pupil needs to be that of cooperators exploring knowledge (rather than that of givers and passive receivers of information) . . .'

(Abercrombie, 1979; cited by Brandes and Ginnis, 1986)

Nurse education is undergoing a major change in the form of Project 2000 (United Kingdom Central Council for Nursing, Midwifery and Health Visiting, 1986). Within this, in keeping with the above remarks, students are encouraged to 'take personal responsibility for their learning' and 'develop their intellectual abilities, self-awareness and self-direction' (English National Board for Nursing, Midwifery and Health Visiting (ENB), 1989). Student-centred learning is a means towards this end, and Bruner's (1966) theory of teaching lends itself as a framework within which to explore this method of learning. Bruner's approach includes learning by problem-solving, discovery methods and inductive reasoning, all of which will be examined further in this chapter using the teaching of nursing care in haematological disorders as the subject example. Bruner (1966) contends that a theory of instruction has four main features.

First it should address *predispositions to learning*, for example, what previous experiences in education and in life would help a person learn to become a nurse? (These could be as diverse as studying Biology at school, giving a basis for further learning to take place, or being a patient in hospital and observing the work of nurses.)

Second, it should state how a body of knowledge should be *structured* so that it can be most easily understood. Bruner looks for the principles and key concepts of a subject to be taught – for example the key concepts for structure and function of blood might be: (a) transport and communication; (b) defence; (c) clotting; and (d) blood groups.

These concepts encompass ideas about relating the structure of the blood components to their function.

Third, effective *sequencing* of the material to be learned is important; for example (a) normal blood, (b) abnormalities, (c) nursing implications. Bruner (1977) favours a spiral curriculum approach, in which a subject is initially presented in a simple form and successively revisited in more complex forms. This is in keeping with the philosophy of Project 2000, in which branch programmes are built upon the Common Foundation Programme to 'provide a continuing educational process' (ENB, 1989).

Fourth, a theory of teaching should specify the nature and pacing of rewards and punishments (*reinforcement*) in the process of learning and teaching. Bruner (1966; 1977) also favours progression towards intrinsic reward, for example the satisfaction of solving a complex problem. This is appropriate to nursing as the practice of nursing demands a problem-solving approach (and students are required to demonstrate this ability) and offers only intrinsic rewards, for example a patient progressing in response to prescribed nursing care.

Knowles (1978; cited by Jarvis, 1983) has formulated a theory of adult learning (andragogy) contending that this can be differentiated from pedagogy on the following assumptions:

(a) adults have a change in self-concept, and need to be more self-directive;
(b) adults have an expanding reservoir of experience which is a rich resource in learning;
(c) adults have a readiness to learn relevant material in order to solve problems in which they are involved; and
(d) adults have a problem-centred, rather than subject-centred, orientation.

Many educationalists would argue that Knowles' theory is invalid as a theory of *adult* learning since his assumptions could equally be applied to children. This point is discussed further in Chapter 7. However, as a theory of learning it is valuable and is of use when considering a student-centred approach. It also has ideas in common with Bruner's theory, in that Bruner (1966) also values a person's existing knowledge and seeks to build on it. The problem-solving approach is again strongly favoured and is very relevant to nursing.

Applying educational theory to practice

This chapter is concerned with how a variety of named teaching methods can be used in the promotion of student-centred learning. Sessions on themes (or key concepts) related to haematological nursing have been identified (e.g. bleeding disorders, immunity) and specific examples of these considered (e.g. thrombocytopaenia, anaemia) in order to draw out, by inductive reasoning, principles which could be applied to a variety of related situations (e.g. other bleeding disorders such as Christmas Disease). The pre-registration learning outcomes set by ENB (1989) for Project 2000 students are designed to 'prepare the nursing student to apply knowledge and skill to meet the nursing needs of individuals and of groups in health and sickness, in a specified area of practice.' In order to apply knowledge the student must first of all have a sound grasp of it, and the work which follows helps the student towards this end.

The subject material used has been sequenced through the five sessions and within each session. Session One examines normal blood, and would be appropriate for teaching in the Common Foundation Programme. Sessions Two, Three and Four look at disordered physiology and could be adapted for use in the Common Foundation Programme or in the branch programmes for Adult Nursing or Nursing the Child. Session Five draws together the previous work and focuses on the nursing implications and may therefore be most suitable for use in the branch programmes though a case could be made for its inclusion in the Common Foundation Programme since the student is to be introduced to the assessment of needs and the planning, implementation and evaluation of nursing care at this stage (ENB, 1989).

A non-threatening learning environment has been aimed for. 'Learning goes well when people feel challenged, and badly when they feel threatened. Whenever a learning task becomes threatening, both adults and children feel anxious, and anxiety interferes with the process of learning. A challenge stimulates people to learn; a threat inhibits them.' (Nicholson and Lucas, 1984). This is particularly important in the case of discovery learning and inductive reasoning where students are encouraged to draw conclusions from their findings, and should not be inhibited by any fear of adverse reactions to 'wrong' conclusions.

Session one: Knowledge of blood

Aim   To enable students to establish their knowledge base in this subject.

Content   Basic ideas and information about the nature and functions of blood.

Method   The suggested method is the *pretest*, an example of which follows.
1. What function of blood can be related to the Activity of Living of Breathing (Roper's model of nursing)?
2. What makes blood so efficient at this function?
3. What are the essential requirements of the body before normal blood can be produced?

4. Where in the body does blood production take place?
5. Which of the granulocytes is particularly concerned with defence against invasion by microorganisms?
6. How is this achieved?
7. Why does blood need to clot?
8. What essential components are required for blood to clot?

Answer guide
1. Transport system for O_2 and CO_2
2. Erythrocytes are present in large numbers, have no nuclei (so more room for Hb molecules), have a biconcave shape which gives a large surface: volume ratio, have a thin covering membrane, bind O_2 loosely
3. Vitamins C, B_{12}, B_6, folic acid
   Minerals, for example iron
   Nutrients, for example fat, protein, carbohydrate
   Intrinsic factor
   Erythropoietin
4. Red bone marrow found in flat bones, irregular bones, ends of long bones
5. Neutrophil
6. Chemotaxis, phagocytosis
7. Prevention of capillary leakage, repair following trauma
8. Normal platelets present in sufficient quantity.

Rationale Davies (1976) defines the pretest as 'any set of related questions, which is given to learners before any formal teaching or instruction takes place', though the pretest may also be used as a method in its own right, not just as a pre-instructional strategy. Pressey (1926; cited by Davis, 1976) found that pretests were useful in directing students' attention to relevant topics.

Used as an introduction to the subject of haematological nursing, the pretest would have two major functions. First it would enable the students to assess their level of knowledge of normal blood, and second it would indicate to them the areas of study most relevant to the work to follow, enabling them to prepare themselves adequately. The pretest also makes use of previous learning on the subject of blood, for example work done at school, and provides an opportunity for the material to be rehearsed, thus enhancing learning.

It is important that the pretest is used in a non-threatening manner if students are to obtain maximum benefit from it. This can be done by ensuring that students understand the purpose of the exercise (which is to establish what they know, rather than emphasise what they do not know), by not taking in the work for teacher marking, and by offering help on an individual or small group basis to any students who find themselves very anxious about their level of knowledge. Again, students should appreciate the need for a sound knowledge base to underpin their nursing practice.

Assessment of Learning Students can use the pretest to establish for themselves what they need to revise or learn for the first time, and then use the test as a post-test to reassess their knowledge. The teacher should be available to help students achieve a realistic level of knowledge, and discourage them from transferring large portions of text into their notes with no real comprehension of the subject, but the teacher is not present in the role of information dispenser. If, on registration, students are to take responsibility for their own continued professional development they will need to develop this habit during their educational preparation, and become confident in their ability to study independently.

Further assessment of the learning accomplished here, and evaluation of the effectiveness of the method will occur in future sessions which will build upon this basic information. This can involve self-assessment and assessment by the teacher.

Session two: Anaemia

Aims The aims of this session are twofold:
(a) To enable the students to identify the needs of the anaemic patient.
(b) To enable the students to identify the reasons for the development of anaemia, and appropriate methods of management.

Content The emphasis of this session is on the role of the nurse, and on helping the students to gain insight into how an anaemic person feels. It is then important for the students to understand the reasons for the occurrence of anaemia, and thus the appropriate action to be taken. Three broad categories can be identified here:
(a) Bone marrow failure (e.g. due to malignancy, aplastic anaemia, drugs)
(b) Unavailability of precursors (e.g. iron, vitamin B_{12}, folic acid)
(c) Congenital disorders (e.g. sickle cell disease, spherocytosis).

Pre-instructional Strategy A springboard question could be used as a pre-instructional strategy to focus students' attention on the symptoms related to severe anaemia and to encourage empathy. An example would be, 'What would it feel like to be very anaemic?'

Methods Many teaching methods could be used here, and some examples follow.

(i) Interview method
This could be used in a variety of ways. For example, anaemic patients could be interviewed, with students being involved in the planning of

the interviews. Ideas could be presented by the students about suitable clinical areas (which could include outpatient clinics) to be approached, and measures to be taken to facilitate patient contact (e.g. preliminary visits, letters). It is unlikely that an adequate number of suitable patients will be found for each student to undertake an interview, so each interviewer will be representing a group of students. To prepare for the interview *group work* could be undertaken (under the guidance of the teacher) to plan suitable interviewing strategies.

Alternative ways of using this method include tape recording or videoing an interview with an anaemic patient for replay in the classroom, or inviting someone (e.g. an outpatient or professional colleague) with a history of anaemia to the classroom to take part in a semi-structured interview with the class. Here the students would have prepared the questions beforehand, but there would also be time for open discussion, with the interviewee's consent.

(ii) Discussion

In each of the above situations the students will have amassed information which may need further structuring. Some students may already have achieved this, for example by using a model of nursing in formulating their questions.

The teacher now acts as facilitator, helping students to establish a link between what they have discovered about the nature of anaemia and the functions of blood, thereby arriving at a definition of anaemia. The nursing implications of their discovery should also be discussed, enabling students to link theory to practice, and this aspect would be covered in greater depth if the work was taking place in a branch programme. In order to ensure participation by each member, the discussion group should not be too large, ideally not more than ten students. This may entail the running of more than one group either simultaneously by different teachers or sequentially by the same teacher. Even with such a relatively small group it is possible for some students to miss the point of the work, and fail to understand why the final definition was reached. One way of avoiding this is to invite students, prior to the discussion, to submit their own definition of anaemia on a named piece of paper, so that the teacher can identify any who are floundering and try to ensure that they reach a correct understanding during the discussion.

(iii) Observation and springboard questions

Having discovered something of the nature of anaemia, it is now necessary to consider the different types, the reasons for their development and their management. In order to do this, students could be given access to microscopes and slides showing normal blood and abnormalities such as aplastic anaemia, megaloblastic anaemia, sickle cells, iron deficiency anaemia. Springboard questions could accompany these, for example:

Why do the (abnormal) erythrocytes look like this?

What makes them function inefficiently?

What can be done to change this situation?

From this work the different types of anaemia can be drawn out, together with the role of the nurse in their management, for example dietary assessment and advice, vitamin B_{12} administration, care of a patient receiving a blood transfusion, health education in sickle cell disease. The role of the teacher is to act as an expert, a resource and a guide to the students, to encourage them to arrive at correct, definitive answers (e.g. vitamin B_{12} injections to treat pernicious anaemia) but also to be imaginative and resourceful, for example when ensuring that an elderly lady receives a diet rich in iron, or a young fashion conscious man with sickle cell disease keeps warm in the winter.

(iv) Computer Assisted Learning (CAL): Blood groups

A CAL programme on this subject would allow students to consolidate their learning at their own pace and in an interesting manner. It gives opportunity for slower students to absorb what can be a difficult topic by revisiting various parts of it. Kirchoff and Holzemer (1979; cited by de Tornyay, 1984) found that CAL benefited learners, whatever their preferred learning style. Enjoyable contact with computers and keyboards will also help any students who have not already done so to become familiar with equipment which is being used increasingly in nursing.

From the CAL programmes on blood groups students can work towards answering the questions: 'What would happen to a patient if he or she was given a transfusion of incompatible blood? 'How are patients safeguarded from this occurring?'

The role of the nurse in ensuring that this situation does not accidentally arise can be discussed, and *role play* can be used to illustrate ways in which it could happen, and how to avoid it. For example, the role play could show two pairs of nurses each checking a bag of blood at the nurses' station. They are then called away to an emergency. One nurse returns, picks up a bag of checked blood, and connects it to the wrong patient, who subsequently collapses and dies. The role play can then be repeated to show the correct procedure with the nurses returning to the nurses' station and going through the checking procedure again from the beginning.

Rationale   This session builds on work the students have already done on erythrocyte structure and function, plus any knowledge of blood groups (e.g. from secondary school) and thus acts as consolidation. It also requires them to utilise basic communication skills which are a component of the Common Foundation Programme. One of the intended outcomes of this part of the course is that students are able to demonstrate communication skills, and having to apply these skills (e.g. in developing open questions for the interviews with anaemic patients) helps students to see their relevance to nursing practice. Also by being involved in constructing the interviews they are learning how to learn which contributes towards the development of 'a sense of personal responsibility and commitment to their continuing professional education and development' (ENB, 1989).

One of the pre-registration learning outcomes required of students by ENB (1989) is 'the identification of health related learning needs of patients/clients . . . and to participate in health promotion.' This process is in action here as students consider the ways in which sufferers of various types of anaemia may be helped, and again involves the use of communication skills. Moreover, in using springboard questions (e.g. 'What would it feel like to be very anaemic') the students are being encouraged to empathise with their patients and attempt to understand fully their needs, from which position individualised nursing care can better be prescribed.

An inductive approach is used in these methods. Students find out examples of the effects of anaemia in order to arrive at the principle of what anaemia is. Similarly, they look at examples of different types of anaemia and ask certain questions in order to arrive at the principles of categorising these disorders and managing and caring for patients. Nicholson and Lucas (1984) maintain that learning requires activity, and this principle has also been applied in the methods selected, students being required to interview, discuss, look at microscope slides and form links with other areas of study.

Bruner (1966) and Knowles both emphasise the importance of using a learner's own experience, and this can be applied by encouraging students to use any personal experience of being anaemic or of being involved in the care of anaemic patients, as well as valuing their existing theoretical knowledge. The methods described also promote creativity, intuitiveness and the development of problem-solving skills, for example in considering the contribution of nurses to the management of anaemic patients. In the case of the provision of an iron rich diet for an elderly lady, for example, there is no standard correct answer for the students to produce so great imagination can be applied in solving the problem.

Assessment of Learning   Students may return to the springboard questions and assess their ability to answer these. Also during CAL students are asked questions which have to be answered correctly before proceeding, thus giving immediate feedback on their level of comprehension. The teacher and the students can assess learning from their interaction during the session (e.g. discussion), and from the students' ability to make deductions, for example about the nursing implications of their discoveries. The use of communication skills and health promotion skills also provides an opportunity for these to be evaluated within a continuing assessment strategy (ENB, 1989) and helps to break down barriers between subject areas. Further assessment of this session takes place during the final session.

Session three: Immunity

Aims   The aims of this session are twofold:
(a)   To enable students to reach an understanding of the vital role of neutrophils in defending the body from infection.
(b)   To enable students to understand the importance of the role of the nurse in caring for a neutropaenic patient.

Content   The content of this session relates to the function of the neutrophils in health, and the severe problems encountered by patients with a very low neutrophil count. Of particular importance here is the great contribution that nurses have to make towards the well-being of these patients. This session will particularly link with the work on the care of patients with leukaemia, but the students will also discover its relevance to the care of any severely immunosuppressed patient, for example those undergoing therapy for certain types of cancer, those with aplastic anaemia, or those who have recently received an organ transplant.

Pre-instructional strategy: springboard question   This could be used as a means of introducing the session and reminding the students of the importance to normal health of the body's immune surveillance system. An example of a suitable springboard question is,
   'What would life be like if you had no neutrophils?'

Methods   Various methods are of use here, and some examples follow.

(i) Buzz groups
Students could be asked to pair up and spend a few minutes preparing a representation of normal neutrophil action (using knowledge from Session One) and also of the effect of having no neutrophils. (Using Bruner's (1977) idea of developing intuitiveness, students may be encouraged to guess at this if they do not know.) This could be presented as a flow diagram, for example as shown in Fig. 5.1, or more artistic students may be able to represent these situations in the form of a series of drawings. Students may require some prompting (e.g. 'What is the worst outcome of infection that you could imagine?') to arrive at the potential seriousness of being severely neutropaenic. Feedback from some students at this stage allows assessment of understanding and correction of any misconceptions within the class.

(i) Normal neutrophil action   (ii) No neutrophils

Bacterial invasion	Bacterial invasion
↓	↓
Chemotaxis	Multiplication of bacteria in blood
↓	↓
Neutrophils move in	Release of toxins
↓	↓
Phagocytosis	Septicaemic shock
	↓
	Rapid death

Fig. 5.1   Example of flow diagrams.

(ii) Market stalls
This exercise requires the assistance of three volunteers (students, or clinical or teaching colleagues) who will need to undertake some preparatory work so that each can man a stall, the teacher manning the fourth. The remaining students divide into four groups (for the four stalls in this example) to rotate around the stalls as follows:

Stall One   Personal cleansing and dressing
Equipment   For example, wash bowl
disposable face cloths
antiseptic and antifungal mouthwashes
pen torch
soft toothbrush

Stall Two   Maintaining a safe environment
Equipment   For example, swabs and culture medium
universal containers
antiseptic handwashing solution
disposable bedpans and bottles
plastic gloves and aprons
picture of domestic assistant

Stall Three   Controlling body temperature
Equipment   For example, temperature recording charts
thermometer
drug prescription chart (antipyretics, antibiotics)
sphygmomanometer

Stall Four   Eating and drinking
Equipment   For example, list of foods to be avoided
photographs of examples of acceptable food
high protein diet sheet
meal replacements/supplements

fluid balance chart
intravenous infusion equipment
drug chart (antiemetics)

These market stalls are based on Roper *et al.*'s (1985) model of nursing and other stalls could be established, for example Eliminating, or Communicating which could have equipment concerned with education and health promotion for the immunosuppressed patient. The students visit the stalls in turn, and use the visual cues and expertise of the stallholder to help them establish, with reasons, appropriate nursing action when caring for a severely neutropaenic patient. Questions could be provided for guidance. For example from Stall Three students see that it is important to measure and record a patient's temperature and blood pressure. They should then be able to apply what they have previously discovered about the consequences of neutropaenia to provide rationale for the selection and suggested frequency of these observations (e.g. a maximum interval of four hours because of the possibility of fatal septicaemic shock).

This part of the session could usefully be summarised by a handout, distributed at the end of the session, and perhaps with sections for students to complete. This would also ensure that the three stallholders did not miss out on information.

Rationale   The springboard question has again been used to focus students' attention clearly on the issue (neutropaenia in this case) which at first sight may not seem a major one as the continuous war which the body wages against microscopic invaders is unseen and unfelt. The buzz groups build on this in a sequential manner and provide a visual representation of the serious consequences of neutropaenia. In the market stall exercise, much room is given for students to work inductively drawing conclusions from the visual cues provided. These visual cues will also be encountered in the clinical area, and some stimulus-response learning may occur here. For example the sight of antiseptic mouthwash in the room of an immunosuppressed patient (the stimulus) may evoke the memory (response) that such patients require very vigilant mouth care in order to minimise the occurrence of mucositis. However, students must also understand the reasons for their actions, not merely perform a ritual, and the stallholders act as facilitators to enable this understanding to be gained. The knowledge gained previously is used to provide a basis for reasoned nursing care.

Assessment of Learning   Students are required to produce something from their buzz groups by which they can assess their own understanding of the function of neutrophils and the implications of their absence. The ability of the students to answer questions posed by the stallholders also provides opportunity for assessment of learning, and evaluation of the methods employed, to take place. The provision of an incomplete handout allows both consolidation of learning (by means of rehearsal) and a chance to assess it, as the students should be encouraged to fill this in without the use of notes or textbooks. This work will be used further, and hence assessed further, in the final session.

Session four: Bleeding disorders

Aim The aim of this session is to help students to appreciate the needs of a person with bleeding tendencies.

Content This session builds on work done on clotting during Session One. Students examine the needs of patients whose blood fails to clot as a result of severely reduced platelet count, absence of clotting factors, anticoagulant therapy or other reasons. The emphasis is on understanding the impact of such disorders on the patient's life, and the role of the nurse in helping the patient to remain well.

Methods Some examples of suitable methods follow, providing a variety of learning experiences for the students.

(i) Diary
Students are asked to imagine that they have some condition which causes them to bleed or bruise following the slightest trauma. They then keep a 24 hour diary, recording any activities which might cause damage to them in this vulnerable state. Students will then arrive for the session with some insight into the problems encountered by the patient with a bleeding disorder and ideas and experiences can be brought together in a plenary session. Some situations which might be observed to hold potential danger are cleaning/flossing teeth, knocking parts of the body, coughing or sneezing violently, spontaneous nosebleeds, sports injuries (major or minor), wounds from kitchen knives or other household tools. A deroling session should be included, in which students are relieved of their imaginary ailment. The teacher can then add, or draw from the students by the use of leading questions, further information about the implications of this state, for example the risk of death from spontaneous cerebral haemorrhage or torrential gastrointestinal bleeding.

(ii) Video
Students may view a video on living with haemophilia. If the diary exercise has already been done, comparisons may be made between situations described on the video and the students' own observations, perhaps giving added interest and relevance to both teaching methods. A video session can be an opportunity for some students to allow their minds to wander, and an accompanying questionnaire to be completed

during the playing of the video can help to overcome this difficulty.

(iii) Group or class discussion
Using the previous material (the diary and the video) students discuss the impact of bleeding disorders on a person's lifestyle, and how they see that nurses can be of assistance in promoting the health of such a person, for example by direct patient care and by education of the patient. (An example of patient education would be to teach the patient to avoid all aspirin containing preparations as aspirin reduces platelet stickiness and irritates the stomach, thus exacerbating the situation.) Afterwards a handout giving examples of the ideas which could be generated during this session will be of use, since students will have little opportunity for note taking during the discussion.

Rationale   The use of the diary method helps students realistically to appreciate the dangers inherent in commonplace daily activities (for example teeth cleaning causes bleeding of the gums if done too vigorously). They are then able to see that they need to apply problem-solving skills to such basic tasks, asking questions such as 'How can oral hygiene be safely and effectively maintained?' The diary also helps to promote the development of empathy in the students by allowing them to 'experience' the difficulties for themselves. The use of the video may provide some welcome input at this stage, after so much student-centred activity, but will also give a useful basis for discussion. Awareness of the discussion to follow may motivate the students to attend and the diary exercise also provides material here.

Assessment of Learning   Some assessment can occur during the discussion period, the teacher being aware of the need to encourage participation by all students, not just by a minority of more vocal group members. This can be facilitated by interacting more directly with any quiet students, for example by asking them for their opinion on something that has been said. Setting ground rules with the class can also prove useful in avoiding domination by a few students. As with previous sessions, this work will also be used further in the final session, giving opportunity for further assessment.

Session five: Leukaemia

Aims   The aims of this session are twofold:
(a)   To enable the students to gain insight into the varying needs of a person with leukaemia.
(b)   To enable the students to understand the value of nursing care for the well-being of such a person.

Content This session addresses the following areas:
(a) The image of leukaemia and reactions to its diagnosis.
(b) The nature of the disease and its management.
(c) The contribution of nurses to the physical, mental and emotional well-being of the patient.

When teaching such a session it is particularly important to be sensitive to the students' reactions and to realise that, for some, leukaemia may have very personal connections, for example a friend or relative may have died from the disease. Such students may feel emotionally unable to deal with looking at leukaemia in the context of a teaching session and may prefer to negotiate alternatives with the teacher.

Methods Some suggestions of usable methods follow. As with other sessions the list is not exhaustive and is offered as a means of stimulating the imagination of the reader.

(i) Brainstorming
This method is used in problem-solving and decision-making (Bligh, 1971) but an adapted version can help to elicit the reactions of the group to the word 'leukaemia', since these are likely to be very similar to the reactions of the general public or a newly diagnosed patient. The teacher could put to the group the question, 'How would you feel if you suddenly found out that you had leukaemia?' or alternatively, if this is felt to be too emotive a question, 'What do you associate with the word leukaemia?' The feelings which emerge may be negative (e.g. death, bald heads, sick children), and these should be recorded (e.g. on flip chart paper) without evaluation for reference at the end of the session.

(ii) Exposition
Some input is required here on the nature of the disease. This could take the form of teacher exposition with contributions from the students, who will have at least some ideas to suggest; for example most will be aware that leukaemia is a malignant disease and has to do with the blood. At this stage a handout would allow students to concentrate without having to write notes. There are other methods which could be used to provide this theoretical input, for example a tape/slide programme or literature searching which could be more student-centred, but some direct teacher contact at this point would help the teacher to assess whether there had been any adverse reactions to the brainstorming exercise, and give opportunity to correct any serious misconceptions about leukaemia (for example the belief that it is still inevitably a fatal disease, or that it is largely a childhood illness).

(iii) Seminars
In order to discuss the disease and its management further, groups of students would undertake to prepare topics for presentation to the rest of the class. These would be short presentations of about 10 to 15 minutes each, and could be on the students' choice of topic, though the teacher may be needed to provide some ideas, for example:
(i)   How is the disease treated?
(ii)   How successful is the treatment and how does this compare with the situation 20 years ago? (Students should be able to demonstrate the tremendous progress made in treatment over this time interval, which helps to put current survival rates for patients with this disease in context. The information could be presented diagrammatically, on flip chart paper or acetate for overhead projection.)
(iii)   What effect does the treatment have on the bone marrow? (Presentation of this information could be enhanced by making available microscopes and slides of normal and treated bone marrow, or projecting slides to show this.)
(iv)   What measures can be taken to support the patient during treatment? (Blood bank may be persuaded to loan to the students out of date packs of blood and platelets, for example, to add visually to this presentation.)
(v)   What are the side effects of treatment and how may nurses help to minimise these? (Students could role play an interview with a 'patient' in remission to present this, allowing subsequent debriefing and deroling for the student who plays the patient.)

Some ideas of the ways in which seminar material can be presented have been included here, but students will often want to use innovative methods of their own. However it is useful for the teacher to be able to help with the provision of suggestions for methods and material if needed. Resources for these seminars include literature (some of which should be available from the teacher) and experts in the subject, for example clinical and teaching staff. The students will also require guidance as to the amount of detail they need, to avoid discouragement if a large volume of material is available. Some students may feel ill-equipped to take part in such a session, and may feel very threatened by having to present information to their colleagues. If the teacher thinks that there is a genuine problem here, it may be preferable to include the student in the group's preparatory work but require minimal verbal contribution, for example introductory or concluding remarks. Feedback to all the students on their presentations should concentrate largely on positive aspects, especially if they have done little of this kind of work previously.

(iv) Role play
Here the students work in groups of three to role play a discussion between a person who has just received a piece of bad news and an

empathic helper, with the third person acting as an observer and taking note of non-verbal as well as verbal interactions. The bad news can be anything which the students choose between them, and may be trivial or more serious as they prefer. After a few minutes of role play, discussion can take place in groups or as a plenary session on how it felt to be in the roles, bringing out both positive aspects and any difficulties which were encountered. The observer will be able to comment on any discrepancies between verbal and non-verbal communication. A deroling exercise must follow this.

(v) Group work: care plans
This work consolidates all the knowledge that the students have already accrued. Students should now be in a position to identify the needs of a person suffering from leukaemia (related to anaemia, immunosuppression and bleeding problems) and give reasoned proposals for the necessary nursing care. Adequate time should be allowed for this (up to two hours) as it is a fairly major undertaking. Students can be facilitated in this work by having on display visual aids which have been used previously, for example items from the market stalls, work produced in the seminars, and relevant literature. The teacher should also make him or herself available as a consultant, and if possible could enlist the help of another expert (e.g. the ward sister or charge nurse) as an additional resource. The role of the expert is as facilitator and guide, not as dispenser of information.

At this stage it is very important for students to take a holistic view of the patient, seeing the interrelationships between all that has gone before. For example it is vital that excellent oral hygiene is maintained in a person who is suffering from leukaemia and has a low neutrophil count, but in making provision for this the fact that bleeding of the gums may occur (due to a low platelet count) must also be taken into consideration.

Rationale   A wide variety of methods has been employed for this final session to help students maintain attention. Bligh (1971) showed that varying the stimuli increased arousal and hence the attention of students, and that long periods (more than 20 minutes) of exposition led to loss of attention. A period of exposition has been included in this section, but with provision for students to contribute what they know or can guess about the nature of leukaemia. This gives opportunity for the students to acquire information which will be essential if they are to appreciate the need of these patients for such careful nursing, but also values what they have to bring from their experience or by intuition as favoured by Bruner (1966; 1977).

The seminar work builds on the exposition, so learners will be able to assess their understanding of the information given and revisit it if necessary. Bligh (1971) finds that seminar work promotes critical thinking in students, which is a necessary skill for the nurse who will find herself in situations where patients' well-being may depend on this. Project 2000 students are also expected to be able to make 'use of relevant literature and research to inform the practice of nursing' (ENB, 1989). This exercise helps students towards this learning outcome since the use of such literature, and literature searching skills, is fundamental to the preparation of the seminars.

The role play is chosen to help students develop empathy and discover that they are able to help people with difficulties or worries. It has been kept as unthreatening as possible, so that no student is put into the emotive position of role playing a patient with leukaemia. The aim is not for students to project themselves into this position, but to realise inductively that such patients will often want someone simply to give them time and space in which to express their feelings, not necessarily to have all the answers. The spiral curriculum is also seen here as students will have had an introduction to communication skills in other areas of the programme and will be applying them here. A plenary session enables students to express any fears they have concerning questions which they may expect to be asked, for example 'Am I dying, nurse?'. It is important for students to understand that not every question has a simple answer, and that they do have something to contribute in such situations. For example, the patient may need someone to acknowledge that they are feeling ill enough to die, and may want to explore the thoughts and feelings that accompany this.

The group work (producing care plans) is a way of rehearsing what has gone before. Bligh (1971) discusses the importance of this in aiding memory, and Bruner (1966; 1977) would see it as holding intrinsic reward for students as they have the satisfaction of bringing together all the threads of the foregoing sessions and producing a useful, meaningful whole. Much problem-solving and inductive reasoning also take place here. As the example of the problem of maintaining a good standard of oral hygiene demonstrates, it is not possible for students simply to work through each session in turn, identifying problems and giving reasoned nursing care. They must bring all of their previous learning to each problem in order to solve it adequately. Project 2000 students are required to have 'the ability to devise a plan of care ...; and (demonstrate) the application of the principles of a problem-solving approach to the practice of nursing.' The care planning exercise helps students to achieve this.

Assessment of Learning   Because of the sequential nature of the exercises, students will be assessing their own understanding of what has gone before as they enter each session. In a non-threatening learning environment they will be free to ask for help or revise previous work as necessary. The production of the care plan from the final exercise is a way of assessing learning, though the teacher will also have to observe carefully to ensure that groups are not carrying passengers who are not participating in the learning. One way to avoid this is to make each group member responsible for leading discussion on one identified area of the care plan.

The teacher may also wish to assess whether there is any change of attitude among the students towards leukaemia. This could be done by producing the results of the brainstorming exercise at the beginning of the session and asking students to form buzz groups to discuss any change in their feelings or reactions towards the disease. One comment could then be taken from each group and the resulting list compared with the original results.

It is clear from the ideas presented in this chapter that student-centred learning is not an easy option for the teacher/facilitator. The quotation at the beginning of the chapter contains within it the idea of a part-nership between teacher and student and, if these methods are to be effective, they must be thoroughly prepared. This may involve more time than is necessary for the preparation of traditional lessons. For example some of the suggested methods involve the acquisition and preparation of equipment, pre-instruction of students and assistants, and planning of interviews. During the sessions themselves the teacher must be on hand as a resource to the students. This implies thorough acquaintance with the subject material, resources and sources of additional information. At times additional help may be required, for example when group work is in progress and there are too many groups for one teacher to visit. If help is unavailable, the teacher could consider running the session twice, with self-directed study (for example use of computer programmes or preparation of seminar topics) running concurrently.

A major benefit of this type of learning is that students are learning how to learn. Using these methods students will gradually become more confident in their own ability to find things out alone, and to solve problems alone or with colleagues. Though they may at first seek reassurance that what they are doing is correct they will move towards greater independence, which can only ease the ultimate transition from student nurse to staff nurse when often there is no one else to provide such reassurance. Furthermore, student-centred learning as described here equips the students with the skills and, it is to be hoped, the desire to learn which will remain with them throughout their professional lives. These attributes are essential if nurses are to keep up to date with current knowledge and research based nursing practice. This is very much in keeping with the stated aims of both the Common Foundation Programme and the Branch Programme in Adult Nursing, in which it is expected that students will develop the ability and motivation to pursue their own professional development (ENB, 1989). Related to this is Bruner's (1966; 1977) idea that rewards should be intrinsic. In the methods suggested in this chapter this is frequently the case. Students are set a question to consider or a problem to solve and suggestions are made as to how they might proceed, but the reward comes from the satisfaction of making progress and reaching a workable solution, not from arriving at a pre-ordained goal.

Finally, at a time of monumental change in nurse education, courage may perhaps be taken from the words of Mark Twain who commented, 'I've foreseen many problems in my life. Luckily many of them never turned up!' (cited by Boud, 1988).

References

Bligh D.A.   (1971).   *What's the Use of Lectures?* Bligh, Exeter.

Boud, D. (Ed.)   (1988).   *Developing Student Autonomy in Learning.* Second edition. Kogan Page, London.

Brandes, D. and Ginnis, P.   (1986).   *A Guide to Student-Centred Learning.* Blackwell, Oxford.

Bruner, J.   (1966).   *Toward a Theory of Instruction.* Belknap Press for Harvard University Press, Cambridge, Massachusetts.

Bruner, J.   (1977).   *The Process of Education.* Second edition. Harvard University Press, Cambridge, Massachusetts.

Davies, I.K.   (1976).   *Objectives in Curriculum Design.* McGraw-Hill, London.

de Tornyay, R.   (1984).   Research on the teaching-learning process in nursing education. *Annual Review of Nursing Research*, **2**, 193–210.

English National Board for Nursing, Midwifery and Health Visiting   (1989).   *Project 2000 – 'A New Preparation for Practice': Guidelines and Criteria for Course Development and the Formation of Collaborative Links Between Approved Training Institutions Within the National Health Service and Centres of Higher Education.* ENB, London.

Jarvis, P.   (1983).   *Adult and Continuing Education: Theory and Practice.* Croom Helm, London.

Nicholson, J. and Lucas, M. (Eds)   (1984).   *All in the Mind: Psychology in Action.* Thames-Methuen, London.

Roper, N. *et al.*   (1985).   *The Elements of Nursing.* Second edition. Churchill Livingstone, Edinburgh.

United Kingdom Central Council for Nursing, Midwifery and Health Visiting   (1986).   *Project 2000: a New Preparation for Practice.* UKCC, London.

Selected bibliography

Allan, P. and Jolley, M. (Eds)   (1987).   *The Curriculum in Nursing Education.* Croom Helm, London.

de Tornyay, R. and Thompson, M.A.   (1987).   *Strategies for Teaching Nursing.* Third edition. Wiley, New York.

Lawton, D.   (1981).   *An Introduction to Teaching and Learning*. Hodder & Stoughton, London. (Studies in Teaching and Learning.)

Quinn, F.M.   (1988).   *The Principles and Practice of Nurse Education*. Second edition. Croom Helm, London.

6 Experiential learning

Linda Smith

Practical aspects of nursing care have been taught experientially for decades and most practising nurses probably remember 'being the patient' while their peers washed, bandaged, lifted and fed them, with varying degrees of skill and gentleness. In more recent years, with the advent of the nursing process, role play and patient-centred group work have been used to teach students such skills as assessment and problem-solving. However, certain areas of the curriculum which could benefit from these methods have often been neglected. One of these areas is the preparation of students for their elderly care experience.

Fielding (1986) showed that negative attitudes towards nursing old people, identified by Robb (1967), still exist today. Her research highlights that the preparation of students for their elderly care experience is often inadequate, with tutorial staff fostering a pessimistic and stereotyped approach to this area of nursing. The description she gives of a preparation which includes wide ranging introduction to the roles of other health care workers, but very little guidance to students about their own role, may be familiar to many readers. Fielding (1986) cites Wells (1980) who suggested that learners were 'a product of a training system that taught them a series of tasks and neglected to provide adequate information about care of the elderly'. However nurses involved with elderly people must be equipped with a depth of knowledge concerning the process and effects of ageing. They should also be helped to develop a positive attitude towards their patients and clients and excellent communication skills, in order to deliver empathic, appropriate and individualised care.

In this chapter a collection of sessions will be presented, all experiential in nature, which may go some way towards assisting the learner to gain knowledge, insight and confidence in the specialty. These sessions embody a philosophy of nursing which emphasises that elderly people have the right to a high standard of individualised, positive medical and nursing care. The time spent caring for elderly people should be seen as just as important an aspect of nurse education as the acute care given on medical and surgical wards and other specialty units which comprise the present pre-registration course for general nurses. The individuality of elderly people should be maintained and they should be helped to overcome the physical, psychological and social difficulties which may arise in old age and to adapt their lifestyle to accommodate the altered circumstances in which they find themselves. This adaptation may enable the elderly person to return to independent life or to accept varying degrees of support which none the less should preserve the identity, dignity, morale and self-esteem of the individual.

The need for nurses skilled in caring for elderly people will increase in the years ahead, for as the United Kingdom Central Council for Nursing, Midwifery and Health Visiting (UKCC) (1985) points out:

'... in terms of demand for services, it is well-known that the population is ageing, and the numbers of very old and frail will be proportionately larger by the turn of the century. Already there are over 8 million people over 65, and by 2001 there will be an additional 0.4 million. As many as 12% of the elderly are likely to be over 85.'

(UKKC, 1985)

These demographic trends undoubtedly present a challenge for nurse teachers responsible for preparing the practitioners of the future. Elderly people, like all clients, deserve the best care possible yet, unfortunately, this specialty is burdened by the twin evils of low professional status and largely negative attitudes within society towards the client group. Furthermore, without exception the nurses are younger than their patients and clients and may hold different beliefs and values. However the radical changes being brought about by Project 2000 (UKCC, 1986) provide an opportunity for a reappraisal of the way nurses are prepared for their elderly care experience, and a key area of the curriculum which should be addressed is the choice of teaching methods.

The sort of issues which need to be discussed with students cannot be dealt with effectively in traditional lecture room settings. Instead the emphasis should be shifted to knowledge gained by experience, knowledge which tends to be remembered and which forms a foundation for further learning.

All human beings learn by and through experience. Thus a person learns much from being part of a situation, but will learn as much, sometimes more, from analysis of the event individually and with others, pondering, reliving and comparing perceptions, to reach acceptable conclusions. From babyhood through to old age, people develop attitudes and values, learn new skills and store knowledge from the constant input of stimuli. Burnard (1985) points out that every acknowledged 'event' adds something to those things that go to make an individual, while Kilty (1982) states that this ability to draw upon experience is inbuilt within the human organism. Nevertheless Pfeiffer and Jones (1980) stress the value of structured experiences, and they argue that 'spontaneous experiences within a group training setting may be valuable in terms of awareness expansion and emotional freedom. However, they may not produce as much personal growth and solid, transferable learning as does a structured experience designed to focus on individual behaviour, constructive feedback and psychological integration'.

In the field of education it would be wasteful not to utilise this natural predilection to learn. Using this style to effect learning is felt, by many educationalists, to be particularly applicable to nursing because so much of a nurse's time is spent in communicating and interacting with others. The provision of relevant situations in which she or he can practise and analyse, build for the future, develop positive attitudes and appropriate intervention strategies in a non-threatening setting can only bring positive results (Kilty, 1982; Burnard, 1985; Miles, 1987). Burnard (1985) describes the concept of experiential learning as having three elements. Involvement in a situation is the first of these. Second, he states that a time of reflection is a vital part of the process to effect learning. Many things happen to us which we do not think about or make any attempt to make sense of. This is an important factor when using such methods as the teacher must ensure that not only is the experience made available, but that the student is given time to reflect upon it. The third element Burnard identifies is the transformation of knowledge into a usable tool on which to build future behaviour. When justifying the use of these strategies Burnard (1985) suggests that this concept and process is valuable in nurse education in that it helps the student towards personal development, including increased self-awareness. It is also of benefit to the learner nurse as it provides the discipline to analyse situations and act appropriately in a variety of settings – a skill essential in the provision of effective care. He calls this 'staying awake' and comments that this reflection requires regular practice in order to become second nature. Finally he maintains that these methods are valuable in the development of nursing skills, particularly interpersonal and empathic skills.

Figure 6.1 shows the concept of the 'experiential cycle' adapted from Miles (1987) in which the steps of review, analysis and synthesis take place. Within this framework Fig. 6.1 shows the four main areas of nursing education which, in the author's view, can be positively affected by experiential learning. It is important that curriculum planners of the future recognise the need for a continuing 'thread' of personal and professional development, because the 'new nurse' must be able to fulfil the aspirations of Project 2000. To do this teachers need to facilitate the development of a nurse who is confident, credible, able to accept accountability and responsibility and who has a sound knowledge-base which she or he can draw on to make decisions about care, in partnership with the patient and the multidisciplinary team.

Experiential learning is a student-centred approach and is the keystone of humanistic education theory. Rogers (1983) asserts that the teacher must be a 'fellow explorer' in the learning process and states that the function of the teacher is to facilitate learning. Certainly each exercise offered will uncover different things for different groups and

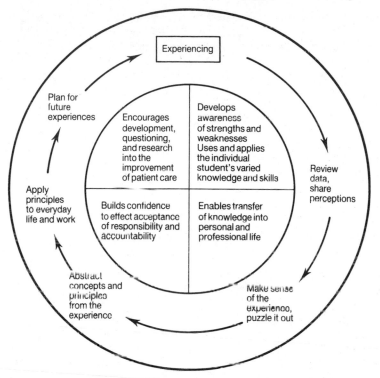

Fig. 6.1 The experiential learning cycle (adapted from Miles, 1987), and the facilitation of personal and professional development in nursing education.

the teacher will learn alongside the students. Nursing students are adult learners and therefore the importance of focusing upon their life, work and academic ability must be stressed. One of the major tenets of andragogy is that learning should be based upon the individual's own circumstances and knowledge (Knowles, 1984). The methods chosen in the following sessions provide a forum in which learners can use their own life events, exercise some choice in what they get out of the sessions and apply their learning to their future allocation in accordance with their needs. The students will have had the opportunity to nurse elderly people during their previous allocations on medical and surgical wards and, in addition, will have friends, relatives and other contacts with elderly people in their life outside work. This experience should be valued and used as a basis for the learning experience offered. Any anxiety or negative feelings which the students may have about their experiences with elderly people should be acknowledged and, wherever possible, alleviated. The students should feel they have access to positive support from both the college of nursing and the service personnel. In using experiential learning methods the reader's attention is drawn to the procedural principles outlined in Chapter 4 (p.116).

Exercises for the development of awareness and insight

It is important that the student has the opportunity to explore his or her own beliefs, values and attitudes towards ageing and the aged. Such views are usually quite firmly entrenched before beginning nurse training but the individual student may not be consciously aware of all of these views, or how they influence behaviour. People will often acknowledge and condemn negative and sometimes harmful prejudice towards others, but still exhibit behaviour that perpetuates it. Dealing with these areas is difficult for the teacher, both from a technical and personal level, so it is not surprising that many teachers prefer to avoid the issues or simply address them from a cognitive stance. An example of this in the case of 'ageism' is the teacher who makes available to the student a multitude of facts, drawn from sociological research into attitudes towards elderly people, in the hope that this alone will enable the students to recognise their own feelings and respond positively to the elderly people in their care. If more than this is attempted when addressing prejudice in any of its forms, then teachers must first have developed the ability to practise honest self-evaluation and have become confident in the interpersonal skills which enable them to deal with any problems which arise. Moreover, a student who is being encouraged to examine and possibly disclose his or her own private internal experience, may require extra guidance and support.

However confident the teacher might be, it is still a potentially difficult area to tackle. In other 'problem' topics of nurse education such as loss, grief, pain, and also certain moral and ethical issues, the student usually has some remembered experience from which to draw parallels and inferences. The experience of being old, however, can only happen when you *are* old and any useful knowledge of it for the young must at best be 'second hand', recounted by someone in the situation. The following exercises might go some way towards providing insight into this normal and, for most, inevitable condition.

Brainstorming

The brainstorming method is an effective icebreaker and instead of being used to promote problem-solving and decision-making (Bligh, 1971) it can be adapted to highlight some of the widely held attitudes towards elderly people. The teacher should write the word 'old' on a flipchart and give the students only a few minutes to call out what comes to mind when they see that word. Their contributions should be included on the flipchart. No discussion of any of the suggested words should be allowed until the class has exhausted all the associative ideas that are generated by the primary word. The technique has been used frequently by the author and almost without exception the response of the class has been negative. For example, 'lonely', 'confused', 'stubborn', 'incontinent', 'wrinkled', 'immobile', 'forgetful' and 'dependent' come up time and again. A few more positive thoughts may be evident in the form of 'grandparent', 'wise', 'loved' and 'leisure', but these are usually much outnumbered by pessimistic ones. The brainstorm can form the basis of a session during which the reality and myths of ageing are examined. The teacher has a wealth of available statistics from sociological research which can be used to show that the stereotyped elderly person is *not* typical and makes up only a small percentage of the elderly population. The concept of the aged person as a biopsychosocial 'whole' being is easily demonstrated by linking the words produced in the exercise under the headings of 'physical', 'sociological' and 'psychological' aspects. Discussions of age-related prejudice, cultural differences, health and well-being and political issues can usually be developed from the exercise and the use of a flip chart will ensure that the brainstorm material can be kept and referred to at the end of the course to evaluate any attitude change.

Guided fantasy

The use of guided fantasy is becoming more popular as a means of developing insight and empathy. The following exercise has been found to be quite effective.

Stage one   The students should be asked to sit in pairs, facing one another. They should then be instructed to look closely at their partners, noting the colour of their hair and eyes, their shape and build, the colour and texture of their skin and the clothing and ornaments they are wearing.

Stage two   The teacher should then ask the participants to close their eyes and imagine they are looking into a mirror. They should be asked to think about what pleases them most about their appearance. Is it a single feature such as eyes or hair, or a combination of features such as figure or face? Time should be allowed for the individuals to think about this.

Stage three   The students should be asked to think about skills or talents which they possess and which please them. Examples could be given such as: Are you athletic? Can you write, draw, sing? Are you articulate or funny or logical? What aspects of your job are best at? What do your partners or friends like best about you? The teacher should then ask the group to try to imagine themselves in a few years time! What do they hope to be doing? What are their ambitions? Where will they be?

Stage four   The group should now be asked to imagine themselves at 70 years old: Where will they be? What changes in their lifestyle may have taken place? What might they have achieved? What would they look like? How would they like people to view them?

Stage five   The students should be told to open their eyes and look again at their partners and try to imagine them at 70 years old. What differences might there be?

Stage six   The students should be directed to tell their partner about one healthy independent elderly person they know. They should describe their appearance, lifestyle, interests and an event in which the elderly person played a part.

The plenary session should involve the whole group and those who wish to disclose any feelings they had should be supported while doing so. The session should end with a tension-releasing exercise or a de-roling exercise in which the group members could be asked to describe something they intended doing later in the day, to ensure that they had accepted the fantasy within the context of their 'real world'. The discussion should be undirected and allowed to range over any aspects that the group wishes, with the teacher only controlling it if an individual exhibits signs of distress or discomfort. It is important, however, that the main points are well summarised and this can be done by the students themselves, with some input by the teacher if necessary.

Paper play

An enjoyable way of illustrating social aspects of ageing and generating discussion is to provide the class with examples of current newspapers and magazines. The students should be asked to form small groups and search the publications for examples of how elderly people are represented. Ageist attitudes, the veneration of youth for its own sake, and the vulnerability of elderly people to crime should be identified easily. In addition, and often to their surprise, the students may find that most news reports about powerful and influential people are, in fact, about people who are of an age which, in western society, is associated with retirement – in the view of many a time of decline into ill health and dependence (Freer, 1988).

Group work

Systemic changes in old age could be used as a focus for group work in which the students would discuss the normal ageing processes and identify how, in certain individuals, adverse consequences may ensue. For example, changes in the urinary system may lead to incontinence, impaired homeostasis and urinary tract infections; cellular changes may lead to delayed healing in an elderly person who has had surgery or suffered trauma. Having looked at the systems in turn the students could then link their conclusions to analyse why elderly people have an increased risk of hospital admission and an increased risk of developing

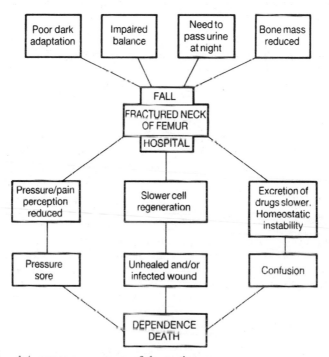

Fig. 6.2. Adverse consequences of the ageing process.

complications whilst in hospital (Fig. 6.2). Finally, the students should suggest ways in which these consequences could be prevented or effectively dealt with by the individual, or the individual and the support team in partnership.

Psychological factors could be used as the basis for discussion about how misconceptions concerning psychological changes in old age may adversely affect the person's mental state and position in society. An effective way of structuring this work is to ask the students to use Maslow's hierarchy of needs (Maslow, 1970) and visualise it not as a triangle but a pyramid. (The students may enjoy constructing an actual pyramid from three triangular pieces of card.) The first facet would illustrate the needs hierarchy, the adjoining facet the possible adverse effects of age, and the third support and intervention to minimise these effects (Fig. 6.3). Finally, learners could discuss physical, social and psychological changes in relation to a model of care.

Handout one: Systemic Changes in Old Age

Cells   Cell division, repair and regeneration is slower. Specialised cells (e.g. ciliated, mucus producing etc.) are often replaced by non-specialised fatty or fibrous cells resulting in a reduction of special function.

Nervous system   The nervous system becomes less efficient generally. Homeostatic mechanisms exert less control. Autonomic impulses may be disturbed. The sorting of sensory data and the subsequent instigation of appropriate action may be less efficient, e.g. balance may be affected. Reflex actions are generally slower (nerve conduction velocity decreases by 0.4% per annum after the age of 60 years).

Cardiovascular system   Cardiac muscle hypertrophies. The valves of the heart become less pliable and the arteries less elastic. Arteriosclerosis and atheroma are commonly seen. The veins are thinner and weaker and the superficial capillaries are unsupported by the ageing skin and therefore easily damaged. The heart of an elderly person does not have the ability to increase heart rate rapidly in response to exercise and then recover quickly as in a younger person. Blood pressure tends to rise in old age mainly due to the increased peripheral resistance caused by the vascular changes.

The urinary systems   There are fewer nephrons in the ageing kidney and up to a 40% reduction in kidney function. The ability to maintain fluid and electrolyte balance is impaired. Bladder tone is reduced and residual urine increases. The autonomic control exerted by the sympathetic and parasympathetic nerves is often disturbed causing irritability of the bladder. The pelvic floor (particularly in women) is weakened and sphincter control is less efficient.

Musculo/skeletal system   Osteocyte regeneration is slower. The inter-vertebral discs atrophy causing loss of height and postural changes. Bone mass is reduced. Calcium leaves the bone due to immobility and reduced oestrogen levels may cause osteoporosis. Vitamin D in the body is often reduced owing to a decreased dietary intake and too little exposure of the skin to sunlight. Joint enlargement occurs and cartilage surfaces fuse together. The muscles lose bulk and power. Sustained effort becomes difficult.

Skin   The skin loses elasticity and subcutaneous fat is reduced. The sweat glands atrophy as do the sebaceous glands. Perception of pain, pressure and heat is reduced by an average of 5%. Hair loss occurs from head and body.

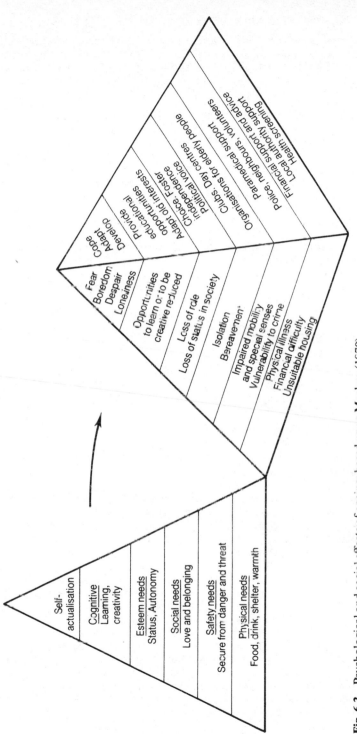

Fig. 6.3 Psychological and social effects of ageing; based upon Maslow (1970).

Respiratory system   The elasticity of the lung tissue is reduced. The muscle power of the chest wall is reduced. Vital capacity shows a marked decrease. The cough reflex is slower and the action of cilia in wafting debris to the surface is less efficient. Accumulation of debris may affect exchange of gases.

Digestive system   Gastric and intestinal motility are reduced. The movement of food through the system is therefore slower. Absorption is less owing to fewer villi in the wall of the small intestine. Less gastric acid is produced and the blood supply to the intestine is reduced. Mucus production is less owing to atrophy of the walls of the gastro-intestinal tract. Insulin production decreases on the whole and it has been estimated that around 60% of people over the age of 70 have clinical or subclinical diabetes. People become 'long in the tooth' as the gums recede. One in three elderly adults have a full set of dentures. Salivary secretion is reduced.

Special senses   The optic nerves may atrophy and cataracts may form. The drainage system of the eye may become less efficient, both internally and externally. Adaptation to dark is reduced or absent. Conductive, occlusive or sensory/neural deafness may occur and most old people experience some impairment of their hearing. The senses of taste and smell become less acute. Pressure, pain and heat perception are reduced.

Reproductive system   The ovaries and uterus in females begin to atrophy when the production of ova ceases at the menopause. Oestrogen production is drastically reduced. The vaginal mucosa is thinner and drier. Breasts lose fat and as a result may become pendulous or very small. In the male, prostatic hypertrophy is common. The male remains fertile for much longer than the female and the ability to have sexual intercourse is unaffected unless there is some other underlying cause. The testes do eventually begin to atrophy and sexual function may wane but men have fathered children when in their eighties.

Handout two: Psychological Factors

Undoubtedly, you will at some point in your nursing careers have discussed how old people change psychologically. Comments about their becoming 'inflexible', 'sad', 'slow of intellect', 'unable to make decisions', 'forgetful' are probably quite familiar to you. However, contrary to popular belief, although these negative changes do occur in some, they are not the inevitable consequences of growing old. The negative feelings which so often occur in relation to getting old are possibly due to attitudes prevalent within our society. 'Ageism' does appear to exist. Elderly people are often underestimated and overprotected and frequently are not 'allowed' to take risks, make decisions, state opinions or preferences 'for their own good'. There is no doubt that some elderly people do have accidents, do make mistakes and do live in poor conditions, which is probably why society has adopted this rather parental attitude towards them, but generalisation should be avoided.

   To compound the problem, a few decades ago psychologists studying the elderly found, in a series of research experiments, that there was a decline in intelligence, a general tendency to withdraw from the world and an inability to learn new material. Psychologists today criticise these findings as it is now clear that the means used to test the subjects were often inappropriate. These conclusions have largely been discounted, but subsequent ones have shown that though intelligence does not decline, speed and reaction time do. This is important to you as nurses because you may have to teach elderly people new skills or explain new concepts to them. All you need to remember is that elderly people may require more time, possibly more repetition, adequate opportunity to practise and a clear link with their lifestyle and past experience.

It is also commonly believed that long term memory in old people is better than short term. Research has not in fact proved this to be *necessarily* so. Short and long term memory, intelligence and learning can be affected but this is not *normal.* Disease, both physical and mental, individual differences and sociological factors usually underlie these changes when they occur.

The idea that people prepare themselves for death by withdrawing from the world is, again, far too generalised. A person may indeed withdraw but it depends on so many individual extraneous factors that it cannot be regarded as an 'ageing process'. However, theories concerning dis-engagement/activity, despair/integrity are interesting because some elderly folk are at one or the other ends of these continua. If carers could identify the reasons for people being at the despair/disengagement points of the continua, they could perhaps facilitate the restoration of a more positive attitude to life and help those elderly persons towards independence once more.

Creativity has also been widely believed to decline with age, as has the ability to plan, to lead and to organise. Einstein, Picasso, Rubenstein, De Gaulle, Churchill and Mao Tse Tung may all have taken exception to this as might former President Reagan, William Whitelaw, Lord Carrington and Virginia Henderson to name but a few!

The message seems clear: the psychological changes that occur with age are relatively limited. They are dependent upon such a variety of factors that few of them could be said to be a normal consequence of age.

The following group work provides an opportunity for discussion of some of the sociological aspects of ageing.

Activity one

(i) Think of a married couple born in 1905. List the major world/ national/economic events they would have experienced during their life. (Don't worry if your history is a bit vague as to dates.) Write the approximate age they would have been during those events.

(ii) Discuss how each of these events might have shaped their lives. Write notes against the list.

(iii) From your own personal experience of elderly people list their *possible* attitudes towards marriage, children, sex, money, politics, youth, work, food, pleasure, entertainment and education. Suggest reasons for these attitudes and *be objective.* Do not be too negative and do not generalise too much. The generation gap works both ways!

Activity two
(i) Think about the losses which are suffered by elderly people. Make a list of all these losses. Now discuss how the individual could come to terms with these losses and write your ideas against the list. Roper (1988) gives 'Dying' as the last of her activities of living. How do you feel about that and why do you think she included this category?
(ii) Have you actually met a sick old person who said 'Why don't you let me die?' If you have, what were the surrounding circumstances? Discuss the 'face to the wall syndrome' where people just seem to give up. Why do you think this happens? Do we really help people to behave positively towards their illness?
(iii) Is there a different attitude to loss and suffering in different ethnic groups? Do you think, for example, an Asian grandparent may suffer less as he or she grows old or do you think there is no difference?

Activity three
(i) Many elderly people suffer from malnutrition. Think of your grandparents or elderly friends and try to list the kind of foods they would consider 'good for you'. Consider fibre, protein, vitamin D, vitamin C, iron, calcium. Make a list of some foods which contain these substances. What would be the consequences of a deficiency of these foodstuffs to elderly people?
(ii) Using your lists, discuss reasons why elderly people often have a diet which is not conducive to health. Think of the elderly person from a biological, psychological and sociological point of view.

Activity four
(i) What are your personal feelings about growing old?
(ii) Discuss how the media represents elderly people. What effect might this have?
(iii) Discuss your feelings about the elderly care allocation.
(iv) Think of 'long stay' elderly patients you have nursed on general wards. Do they have special needs? Are these needs met?

These group activities can highlight the myths surrounding ageing as well as the facts, and can lead to a discussion of the many ethical issues which arise when caring for elderly people. If all the activities are to be used then a whole day may be required to allow adequate time for feedback and the expansion of points from the learners' contributions. However, when time is at a premium the use of just one of the activities as part of a shorter session can be effective. In order to ensure that all the students have the opportunity to contribute there should be about four to five people in each group.

Fieldwork

The following fieldwork is designed to help learners gain insight into the practical difficulties experienced by disabled elderly people.

The fieldwork takes a whole day as the feedback can take at least two hours.

Students go in groups of four or five to a shopping centre of their own choice. Each group is given a pack containing various 'props' to simulate disablement if they so wish (earplugs, wheelchairs, doctored spectacles etc.). The members of the groups will undertake to ensure that their colleagues come to no harm if they choose to wear the disabling devices.

Some suggested observations for each group

1. Count the public lavatories available. Note their type and suitability for elderly people.
2. Note the number of benches available.
3. Are the public transport facilities appropriate for the elderly population?
4. Do major stores have lifts, escalators, stairs only?
5. Stand in a busy part of the street, count a hundred people and estimate the percentage of elderly people who shop there.
6. Are there *suitable* refreshment places for elderly people?
7. How many shops cater for elderly people, e.g. shoe shops, clothing shops?
8. Are there any leisure facilities for elderly people? Check out the library, parks, clubs.
9. Note special problems of elderly people from other ethnic groups.

The exercise has, without exception, generated amazement among students that something which they take for granted, such as shopping, should be so difficult and frustrating when even mild physical problems are present. Lively discussions on design and attitudes have invariably ensued and if the learners have visited different shopping centres, comparisons have been possible. Unsafe surfaces, public transport provision, poorly designed entrances and exits to buildings and inadequate toilet facilities are aspects of daily living which have been identified by students as a cause of distress to people whose sight, hearing or mobility is impaired.

Day room

The aim of this session is to help students to identify problems in ward design, communications and management which may be experienced by both patient and nurse in an elderly care unit.

Role play

The students should be asked to pretend they are 'patients' in a day room attached to an elderly care ward. The chairs should be arranged round the room against the walls. A small group should be sitting round a table or coffee table, facing one another, in a more intimate setting. Three volunteers should be sought to play the nurses and two volunteers to observe the proceedings. (Students who do not wish to 'play' could perhaps take on this role.)

'Props' required   Spectacles for the sight impaired patients, ear plugs for deaf patients, knitting, book, walking frame, box of smarties or similar small sweets.

The patients should all be given a role to play from the list. They can develop the role as the circumstances demand but should be asked to try to achieve the goal suggested by the role, for example go to the toilet, get a cup of tea. The nurses should be told that they can care for the patients as they see fit but during the exercise each of them must leave the room once and stay away for four minutes in order to complete a task, for example, answer the phone, see the doctor etc. In addition, a 'medicine round' must be completed. Two smarties are to be given to each patient (the checking routine may be omitted) but if any patient makes a query or expresses concern, this should be dealt with. Anything else that happens should be managed as the nurses wish. None of the nurses is senior to the others. The patient roles are as follows:

Role one   You are Mrs Andrews. Your hearing is poor and you are waiting for your daughter to come and tell you how your husband is getting on alone at home. He is rather unsteady on his feet and can't visit you himself. You are quite anxious because she is late.

Role two   You are Mrs Allison and you believe that the tablets that the nurses give you are poisonous. You think they are keeping you a prisoner and you want to escape. You can walk.

Role three   You are Mrs Jones. You cannot see well. You want to go to the toilet. You're afraid you'll wet yourself.

Role four   You are Mrs English. You are going home tomorrow but you are worried about your new tablets. You want to know what they do. You know they are 'water tablets' and 'heart tablets'.

Role five   You are Mrs Johnson. You are quite happy because you are getting better and will be going back home in a few days. You'd like to watch the television but it has a notice saying 'Ask the staff to switch T.V. on if you wish to view'

Role six   You are Mrs Bowden. You dislike being in hospital and your bottom is sore. You can't walk but to ease your bottom you decide to slide off the chair.

Role seven　You are Mrs Smith. You want to go back to your bedside to get your photograph album. You can walk with a zimmer frame.

Role eight　You are Mrs Ayton. You can't remember where you are but you know you must go and do some shopping and you decide to do it now.

Role nine　You are Miss Sullivan. You are trying to read your book and people will not let you concentrate. You like being on your own.

Role ten　You are Mrs Walton. You are quite happy but they have put you some distance away from your friend, Mrs English. You have to be helped to walk over to her.

Role eleven　You are Mrs Parker. You would love a cup of tea and you are wondering if the nurses will make one for you.

Role twelve　You are Mrs Porter, who will be going to a home. You do not mind but you forgot to ask the social worker whether you could still claim your pension. You decide you'll ask the nurse when she comes round.

Role thirteen　You are Mrs Singh. You do not speak much English. You want to know if your son has telephoned because his wife is due to have a baby soon. It's your first grandchild. You are pleased and excited.

Role fourteen　You are Miss Caldwell. Your ball of knitting wool has rolled away. You'd like the nurse to pick it up and attach a carrier bag to your chair to put it in so it can't roll any more.

The enactment of this exercise and the subsequent discussion are likely to be quite lively as the activity is partly designed to highlight frustration. Deroling of all participants should take place. However, if the teacher is concerned that a particular group might find any of the roles difficult or might overact a little, the more difficult roles can be omitted or played by another teacher. The teacher might like to play the ward sister who gives a brief report on the people in the day room (omitting their special desires but including things like 'she's going home', 'she's a bit confused at times') and then tells her 'new students' she'll be busy elsewhere and unavailable for questions!

The feedback varies with whatever happens in the role play, but in the author's experience students are likely to discuss feelings of frustration, the importance of comprehensive reporting, the need to know one's patients, the problem of differing priorities for staff and patients and the layout of furniture in communal areas.

Confusion

The following simulation is intended to give students some insight into how it might feel to be confused and is envisaged as part of a longer session relating to reality orientation. It requires much cooperation from the students, and a teacher who is able to talk nonsense without laughing or becoming embarrassed. Some examples of 'nonsense' are given on the following pages but teachers may wish to use other material with which they feel happier. The simulation requires about 15 minutes. The nature of the simulation is such that it tends to get 'ragged' if more than this time is taken. The discussion and debriefing take much longer, however, and in the author's opinion *at least* an hour should be given to the whole session. It is an advantage if two teachers can facilitate this exercise together since it is important to be alert to any signs of distress among the students. In addition careful deroling of all participants is essential.

The students should be asked to sit in their chairs in a circle. There should be plenty of space surrounding the circle, so desks should be stacked away. The students who wish to participate should be asked to put on a blindfold.

NB   It should be stressed to the students that confused people are not necessarily blind but that the suppression of one of their senses will help them to gain insight into the problem. The effect sensory loss has on the mental state of the patients can be developed later in the discussion.

When the students are settled and blindfolded, the teacher should give the following instructions:
If a sentence is preceded by the word 'Right' it is a real instruction and they can do whatever is asked.
If a sentence is preceded by the words 'Listen carefully' the students should try to remember as much as they can about the words that follow.
No further communication should be acknowledged even if the students ask questions.
Maintain silence for at least 2 minutes.
Walk round the room allowing the students to hear you make noises if you wish. (You could, for example search noisily in a box or a cupboard.)
Lightly touch *some* of the students as you pass. Do not respond to any shocked reactions. Deliberately ignore a few students; do not touch them or move close to them.
Move the students round. Change them from chair to chair. Leave some standing in the middle of the room. Give explanations to some and be uncommunicative and hurried with others.
Eventually finish by sitting them all down again in different chairs. Say 'Listen carefully' and then read a passage from a book. It should be quite detailed to have a good effect in the ensuing feedback. (The author has used poetry and passages of fiction and non-fiction.) Maintain silence following this passage. A repetitious noise could be introduced

after a minute or so. (The author rolled a pen over the desk.) Then read a news report without the words 'Listen carefully' preceding it:

Runaway train crash

British Rail launched an investigation yesterday after a train careered backwards out of control for more than two miles before smashing into another train moments after all the passengers had got off.

No one was injured in the collision between the runaway mail train and an empty passenger train near Liss station, Hampshire, on the main London to Portsmouth line.

Seventy-four cups of tea were spilled in the collision between the empty dustbin and the runaway mail train in Hampshire yesterday. Many people avoided the air-raid by hiding under a herd of sheep and a cat which they found on the line. A spokesman reported that the driver would not have become unconscious had the Government's plan to poison all nurses by giving them dangerous tablets been carried out as promised.

Twelve hours after the smash the line was still blocked as accident investigators visited the scene.'

Try not to change your tone when reading this. Teachers might like to 'doctor' their own news report, but to be effective the report should contain a proportion of ridiculous or nonsensical phrases.

If you have a partner you could then hold a whispered conversation using the names of some of the students. Finish with the words 'Let's get it then', walk to the door and open and close it, then just wait quietly for a few minutes.
Say '*Right* – you can take your blindfolds off and open your eyes now'. You will probably find you need to repeat this instruction.
End exercise.

The feedback will probably include the students' feelings of uncertainty, anxiety and anticipation of the next event. Some feelings of anger may be expressed at the vague instructions. The students usually remember a good deal about the first passage which is likely to surprise them. The news report, however, will probably not be remembered so well, apart from the nonsense. The discussion could focus upon the need for clear instructions and repetition and how misheard or badly phrased communication could be a source of distress. The teacher could point out if necessary how a distant conversation, television or radio in the background could possibly fix an idea in the mind of a confused person or even establish a paranoid delusion. Following the discussion the teacher should become quite business-like and tell the class they will now look at the causes of confusion and dementia. Ask the class to copy down the definition on the overhead projector transparency slide (Fig. 6.4) as this is a good summary of the condition. Switch on the

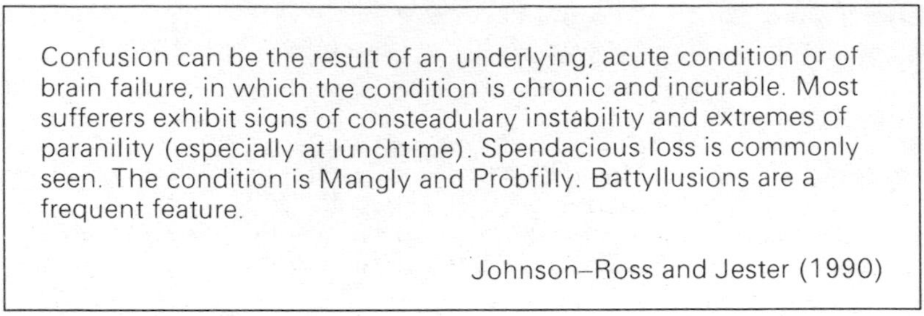

Confusion can be the result of an underlying, acute condition or of brain failure, in which the condition is chronic and incurable. Most sufferers exhibit signs of consteadulary instability and extremes of paranility (especially at lunchtime). Spendacious loss is commonly seen. The condition is Mangly and Probfilly. Battyllusions are a frequent feature.

Johnson–Ross and Jester (1990)

Fig. 6.4 'Nonsense' overhead projector slide to illustrate difficulties experienced when ability to interpret the written word is lost.

projector *after* these instructions have been given. The students will probably write a few sentences before 'catching on' and the last part of the discussion could centre upon the experiences of people who can no longer decipher written instructions and the effects this might have.

Equipment box

The equipment box described below can be kept by the teacher for use whenever appropriate. The various disabling devices can be used as part of specific sessions previously mentioned or just used by the students as they go about the school or hospital. For example effective learning has been achieved by students' just wearing ear plugs to the dining room. Some suggestions for the contents of the box are listed. Teachers may find other equipment such as walking aids, aids for eating and drinking and articles of clothing with zips, buttons and velcro fastenings useful. Hearing aids can be included but the author suggests they are only used to demonstrate cleaning, fitting and battery changing as the indiscriminate use of the aid to magnify sound can cause damage to the student's hearing. Some useful 'props' could be as follows: disposable wax ear plugs; spectacles which have been sandpapered (very poor sight) or painted with an irregular black 'splotch' in the centre of the lens (cataract) or irregular spots (macular degeneration); swimming goggles painted black (blindness); wrist splints (which should be incorrectly applied to achieve disablement) (Fig. 6.5); neck collars; knitting; a 'tinnitus' tape to be used with personal stereo sets (easily produced by taping a continuous noise, whistles, machinery etc. – the author used a garden strimmer!); bandages for blindfolds; some childproof medicine bottles and other household items

Safety rules must be agreed when the students use the 'props'. Students should be given complete choice about whether they use these 'props'.

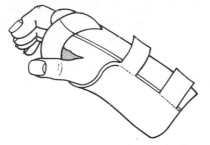

Fig. 6.5 Diagram to show how a misapplied wrist brace can be used as a disabling device.

Evaluation of the sessions

Though some students inevitably find these methods threatening, on the whole they appear to be effective. Student evaluations collected by the author have stated that the exercises helped them understand the problems of elderly people, took the fear out of the elderly care allocation, made them examine their own attitudes and helped them to see patients as biopsychosocial individuals. The methods have also been successfully tried with groups of post-registration students, some of whom were older, traditionally trained sisters, and with local authority care assistants. These more experienced groups were surprisingly enthusiastic and brought a new perspective to discussions and feedback. However, the sessions require time and meticulous organisation and, in spite of this, some of the exercises, notably 'day room' and 'confusion' can get out of hand, with much overacting and laughter. Nevertheless, in the author's experience, even when this has happened, the issues have still been recognised. With regard to this it is crucial that students are always helped to work through the experiential learning cycle (Fig 6.1, p.147).

No formal, structured evaluation of clinical practice has yet been attempted, so it is unknown whether the new style has had any direct effect upon patient care. However, post-experience evaluations have seemed more positive since the introduction of these approaches.

The reader should note that the experiential components of the curriculum 'thread' can be supported by more formal teaching in other aspects of care such as the roles of other members of the multidisciplinary team, disease-related topics and specific 'problem' areas such as incontinence, abuse of elderly people and pharmacology. Curriculum planners should consider this 'thread' in the context of Project 2000 and the demographic trends which suggest that a large percentage, and possibly a majority, of patients/clients cared for by those students who opt for Adult Nursing will be elderly. (This must, of course, include

the Mental Health and Mental Handicap Branches.) It is interesting
that UKCC (1986) envisaged that the Common Foundation Programme would contribute to bringing about changes in professional
values and attitudes towards elderly care, by 'giving all practitioners an
initial acquaintance with the needs of elderly people, with the challenges
of providing care for them, and with examples of improvements in
practice in this key field'.

Sick elderly people are *sick adults* and should not be seen as members
of a race apart but be integrated into the health care network, whether
they receive treatment in elderly care units or general wards. They are
adults, however, who may have other age-related problems which nurses
should learn to recognise and plan for from the beginning of their
educational programme. As the World Health Organisation (1978)
suggests, 'care for the elderly in hospital and community settings
requires, among other things, a thorough knowledge of the process of
ageing and of the psychological, sociological and health-orientated
aspects of care, indeed, of its person-orientated rather than disease-
orientated aspects'.

It is painful to reflect that, in spite of the recognition of shortcomings
and inequalities in the care of our elderly sick people over the last two
decades, very little has in reality changed. The curriculum *still* does not
provide adequately for this branch of nursing in many centres of learning and nurses are still exhibiting negative responses. It is the teacher's
duty to try to redress the balance and facilitate the development of
more positive attitudes in the nurses of the future.

References

Bligh, D.A.   (1971).   *What's the Use of Lectures?* Bligh, Exeter.
Burnard, P.   (1985).   *Learning Human Skills: A Guide for Nurses.*
    Heinemann, London.
Fielding, P.   (1986).   *Attitudes Revisited.* Royal College of Nursing, London.
Freer, C.   (1988)   Old myths: frequent misconceptions about the elderly. In
    The Ageing Population: Burden or Challenge? N. Wells and C. Freer (Eds),
    pp 3–15. Macmillan, Basingstoke.
Kilty, J.   (1982).   *Experiential Learning.* Human Potential Research Project,
    University of Surrey, Guildford.
Knowles, M.   (1984).   *The Adult Learner: A Neglected Species.* Third
    edition. Gulf Publishing, Houston, Texas.
Maslow, A.H.   (1970).   *Motivation and Personality.* Second edition. Harper
    and Row, New York.
Miles, R.   (1987).   Experiential learning in the curriculum. In *The
    Curriculum in Nursing Education*, P. Allan and M. Jolley (Eds), pp 85–
    125. Croom Helm, London.
Pfeiffer, J. and Jones, J.   (1980).   *Structured Experience Kit: Users Guide.*
    University Associates, San Diego, California.

Robb, B. (1967). *Sans Everything: A Case to Answer*. Nelson, London.
Rogers, C.R. (1983). *Freedom to Learn for the 80s*. Charles Merrill, Columbus, Ohio.
Roper, N. (1988). *Principles of Nursing in a Process Context*. Fourth edition. Churchill Livingstone, Edinburgh.
United Kingdom Central Council for Nursing, Midwifery and Health Visiting (1985). *Project 2000: Facing the Future, Project Paper 6*. UKCC, London.
United Kingdom Central Council for Nursing Midwifery and Health Visiting (1986). *Project 2000: A New Preparation for Practice*. UKCC, London.
World Health Organisation (1978). Summary report of a working group on nursing aspects in the care of the elderly. *Journal of Advanced Nursing*, **3(4)**, 407–12.

Bibliography

Adams, G.F. (1977). *Essentials of Geriatric Medicine*. Oxford University Press, Oxford.
Anderson, W.F. *et al.* (1982). *Gerontology and Geriatric Nursing*. Hodder and Stoughton, London.
Baker, D.E. (1983) 'Care' in the geriatric ward: an account of two styles of nursing. In *Nursing Research: Ten Studies in Patient Care*, J. Wilson-Barnett (Ed.), pp 101–17. Wiley, Chichester.
Bergman, R. and Golander, H. (1982). Evaluation of care for the aged: a multipurpose guide. *Journal of Advanced Nursing*, **7(3)**, 203–10.
Boyd, R.V. (1981). What is a social problem in geriatrics? In *Health Care of the Elderly*, T. Arie (Ed.), pp. 143–57. Croom Helm, London.
Brocklehurst, J.C. (Ed.) (1978). *Textbook of Geriatric Medicine and Gerontology*. Second edition. Churchill Livingstone, Edinburgh.
Carver, V. and Liddiard, P. (Eds) (1978). *An Ageing Population*. Hodder & Stoughton in association with the Open University Press, Sevenoaks.
Entwistle, N. (ed.) (1985). *New Directions in Educational Psychology 1: Learning and Teaching*. Falmer, London.
Hanley, I. and Gilhooly, M. (Eds) (1986). *Psychological Therapies for the Elderly*. Croom Helm, London.
Holden, U.P. and Woods, R.T. (1982). *Reality Orientation: Psychological Approaches to the Confused Elderly*. Churchill Livingstone, London.
Isaacs, B. and Evers, H. (Eds) (1984). *Innovations in the Care of the Elderly*. Croom Helm, London.
Jorm, A.F. (1987). *Understanding Senile Dementia*. Croom Helm, London.
Lovell, R.B. (1982). *Adult Learning*. Croom Helm, London.
McHeath, J.A. (1984). *Activity, Health and Fitness in Old Age*. Croom Helm, London.
Wade, B. (1983). Different models of care for the elderly. *Nursing Times*, Occasional Papers, **79(12)**, 33–6.
Webb, C. (1981). Classification and framing: a sociological analysis of task-centred nursing and the nursing process. *Journal of Advanced Nursing*, **6(5)**, 369–76.

7 Independent studies and the curriculum in nursing education

Alan Myles

Introduction

This chapter will first explore the nature of independent studies with reference to the tenets of andragogy and Bradshaw's (1972) concept of social need. Second, an account of different modes of independent study and their place in nursing curricula will form the substance of the text. The principles and practice of open/distance learning, contract learning, and elective options as exemplars of independent study will be discussed. Finally, some of the wider implications of an increased emphasis on independent study in nursing education will be addressed.

The concept of independent study

Independent is defined as 'free from the influence or control of others; self-governing; self-confident; self-reliant' and also as 'a person who is independent in thinking, and action' (Collins, 1981). Studies have been defined as 'the application of the mind to acquire knowledge, as by reading' (Collins, 1981). The notion of developing one's knowledge in an autonomous way may seem on the one hand attractive in that individuals can pursue that which interests them. On the other hand, should learning for a profession which requires that its members are safe and competent to deliver individualised nursing care in a variety of settings be totally free from external influence? Perhaps the concept of *interdependent study* is a more appropriate one. In this chapter the concept of independent study will be regarded as 'a predominantly self-regulating mode of broadening one's knowledge and skills'. This precept will be further developed with reference to the tenets of andragogy.

Andragogy

Andragogy has been defined as the art and science of teaching adults as compared to pedagogy, the art and science of teaching children (Knowles, 1984). The author argues whether it is a science as yet. For example, is there sufficient empirical evidence upon which to substantiate that claim? Other writers suggest that it is an ideology rather than a theory of adult education and that it is a term given to an expanding body of knowledge of how adults learn (Mezirow, 1981; Jarvis, 1983).

Knowles can be regarded as the 'father' of andragogy and differentiates andragogy from pedagogy on five assumptions (Knowles, 1984).

1. Self-concept Knowles argues that adults are more self-directing, whereas children are more dependent on the teacher for decisions about their learning. This is not necessarily the case since many children are quite capable of negotiating their own learning needs. Nevertheless, the point about adults taking more responsibility for their own learning is well made, a principle compatible with the concept of independent study as previously defined.

2. Role of experience Knowles argues that adults have a vast reservoir of experience which can be drawn upon during the learning process as opposed to a child's more limited experience. This is also suspect since the experience of children can be incorporated into teaching sessions. However, the point about using the students' experience (adult or child) is worthy of reinforcement, and apposite to the current discussion in that individuals can build on their reservoir of knowledge through independent study with guidance if required.

3. Readiness to learn Knowles argues that an adult's readiness to learn becomes orientated increasingly to the developmental tasks inherent in his or her social roles. It can be argued that this also applies to children, but the essential point here is the importance of relevance. Independent study is likely to fulfil this criterion since individuals are unlikely to pursue subjects that hold no relevance or interest for them.

4. Orientation to learning The assumption here is that a pedagogical curriculum is subject-based whereas an andragogical curriculum should be problem-based. The author believes that this assumption can be dismissed with reference to Beattie's (1987) fourfold curriculum in that a curriculum for adults or children could be based on a map of key subjects, schedule of basic skills, portfolio of meaningful experiences, and an agenda of important cultural issues. Independent study can also be based on the tenets of the fourfold curriculum. This point will be further developed and illustrated with practical examples later in the chapter.

5. Motivation to learn   It is asserted that the essential difference is the source of motivation, i.e. extrinsic for children and intrinsic for adults. Again, this assumption can be dismissed in that the author believes that both adults and children are motivated extrinsically and intrinsically. The important point here is that teachers need to try and foster intrinsic motivation, and (almost paradoxically) extrinsic motivation can achieve this. For example, encouragement and praise can develop a student's interest in a subject. The concept of intrinsic motivation is clearly an important aspect of independent study, but the potency of extrinsic motivation should not be overlooked. This point will be illustrated during the discussion on open and contract learning.

To summarise thus far, it can be stated that the assumptions upon which pedagogy differs from andragogy are suspect. However, the tenets of andragogy can be regarded as principally axiomatic. It is currently a favoured ideology in nursing education, reflected by a growing interest in the area of independent study. This premise will be further developed with reference to Bradshaw's (1972) concept of social need.

Social need

Bradshaw (1972) argues that social service is based on need of which he describes four types: normative, comparative, felt and expressed. Normative need is what the expert or professional defines as need in any given context. The content of sessions chosen by teachers can be regarded as normative in that it is based on professional expertise and judgment. The pre-registration learning outcomes outlined in the English National Board for Nursing, Midwifery and Health Visiting (ENB) Project 2000 guidelines (ENB, 1989b) can be regarded as normative since they suggest the 'desirable standard' to be reached by students to enable them to be admitted to the professional register of the United Kingdom Central Council for Nursing, Midwifery and Health Visiting (UKCC). In the context of independent study, the learning objectives found in the units of an Open University Course can be regarded as normative since they have been devised by the course team.

Comparative need is a measure of need found by studying the characteristics of those in receipt of a service and comparing what type of 'service' different groups receive. In the context of independent study, students may compare the amount and type of support they receive and some may feel they compare unfavourably. Students may feel that an excessive amount of independent study is a 'cop out' by the teaching staff. Felt need is equated with wants and is influenced by perception and motivation, for example the need for a degree qualification.

Expressed need is felt need turned into action. Expressed learning needs can be fulfilled via the various modes of independent study. The first mode to be considered will be open/distance learning.

Open/Distance learning

The terms open and distance learning require clarification. Quinn (1988) describes open learning as a flexible approach to learning which is characterised by student-centredness, using multimedia learning materials, with tutorial support and guidance. He identifies *access* and *control* as two of the most important aspects of open learning. The Open University has a long tradition of accessibility, 'opening its doors' to a large number of the population without the normal university matriculation requirements. The openness refers to the removal of barriers and the facilitation of access to education programmes. The 'centre' is the student, not the educational establishment.

The notion of control can be discussed with reference to Bernstein's (1975) concept of framing. Framing refers to the degree of control exercised over the organisation, pacing and timing of curricular content and processes. Weak framing is characterised by a great deal of student control over learning whereas the converse is true of strong framing. Open learning is clearly an example of weak framing in that the student can decide *what* to study, *when* to study, *how* to study, and *what* to do next.

Distance education is planned on the geographical separation between students and teachers (Quinn, 1988). Students arrange for the receipt of learning materials through the mail which are subsequently 'worked through'. The materials are often arranged in units of study which may be supplemented by radio broadcasts and television programmes. There may also be telephone communications with tutors where students can discuss the units and clarify understanding. Students may also come together in a 'Summer School' and enjoy the benefits of group discussion found in institution-based education. The British Open University is one of the finest and well-known examples of distance education and it is suggested that its principles of distance learning can be incorporated into the education of nurses at both pre and post-registration levels. Also, the Distance Learning Centre (DLC) at London's South Bank Polytechnic produces excellent materials specifically for nurses. A range of units of study are available including a 'user friendly' series on research.

Holland (1989) states that the uptake of open and distance learning has had a 'disappointingly sluggish start' in nurse education. Perhaps this is not surprising if the introduction of open and distance learning was perceived by some potential users as via an empirical-rational strategy of change. According to Bennis and others the belief under-pinning the empirical-rational strategy is that people are guided by reason and that they will employ a rational calculus of self-interest in determining needed changes in behaviour (Bennis *et al.*, 1976). The empirical-rational approach assumes that knowledge is a source and ingredient of power. Knowledgeable people are power holders, and desirable change is effected through the transfer of knowledge (power), in the education process, to those who lack the specific knowledge (ENB, 1987). It can be argued that the designers of open/distance learning materials are the 'power holders', and that the target population, i.e. the intended users, are those who need the 'knowledge' in those materials. Holland reinforces this point by referring to the belief held by some tutors that the open/distance learning materials produced by larger institutions do not address local differences and needs (Holland, 1989). She goes on to state that other tutors and managers also have problems in appraising existing materials effectively and have not worked out how to adapt materials to suit the local situation. Through the experience of facilitating a wide range of work-shops for different teacher groups based on open learning materials, the author suggests that users are now more creative at selecting and adapting components to meet their needs (it should be stressed that this observation is offered with a degree of humility). The reason for this perceived uptake in the use of open/distance education is probably due to a variety of reasons which include:

- wider range of relevant quality materials available on the market;

- developmental testing 'sensitises' users to their use;

- demands of Project 2000 encourage groups to manage change through the shared use of open learning workshop materials;

- facilitators are being invited to run workshops and help users to adapt the materials to meet their local needs; and

- the increasing popularity of contract learning (a mode of open learning it could be argued).

Holland (1989) suggests that enthusiasm to both use and produce materials at local level should be encouraged. She goes on to warn of the dangers of enthusiasm alone being insufficient to ensure the rigorous quality control needed to make open learning materials credible. The author is familiar with the following stages which need to be 'worked through' to produce quality open learning materials.

Stage 1   Identify needs of potential users
This activity could be carried out initially by members of one of the statutory bodies. For example 'Preparing for change' was part of a

three year ENB project aimed at helping nurse teachers and senior education managers respond to the major changes facing the nursing profession (ENB, 1987). This reinforces the ENB's commitment to open/distance learning as an important means of supporting the continuing education of nurses, midwives and health visitors.

Stage 2   Form a Working Group

A working group is formed whose membership should reflect the needs of the potential users. In 'research language' they should be a representative sample of the target population with additional expertise as needed, for example professional learning materials designers. The working group works on the:

● aims and audiences

● content and structure

● interactivity, i.e. various modes of engaging the users in activity

● mode of use

An important aspect of this stage is the identification of contributors, i.e. writers. It is imperative that contributors are fully briefed as the preparation of open learning materials is different from writing chapters for textbooks or articles for journals. For example, writers must ensure that users will have sufficient opportunity to 'engage with the text' through a range of individual/group activities. Contributors may emerge from the working group as well as from outside.

Stage 3   Draft One materials are produced

Contributors start work on first drafts which are submitted to the working group who act as critical readers. The fate of first drafts may be one of the following:
 (i)   they are 'binned', i.e. deemed unsatisfactory
 (ii)   they are accepted conditional on modification
 (iii)   they are accepted as a draft two

Stage 4   Draft Two materials are assessed

On receipt of draft two materials, the working group critically reads those materials, assessing their suitability for piloting with a representative sample of the user group. Following this activity materials are sent out for use.

Stage 5   Developmental testing

The open learning materials are tested during this phase and feedback is given to the working group. The feedback will lead to one, some, or all of the following:
 (i) draft twos are 'binned'
 (ii) draft twos are modified

(iii) draft twos are accepted for final drafting
During this very important stage, the working group and learning material designers are dependent on the goodwill and commitment of members of the developmental testers.

Stage 6   Production of final version
During this phase most of the working group 'breathe a sigh of relief' whereas the learning material designers face publication deadlines.

Stage 7   Dissemination
The dissemination and uptake of open learning materials may be promoted through official launches and 'roadshows' facilitated by members of the working group.

Following dissemination, the materials may need further improvement and updating. Summative evaluation should be conducted to establish the overall effectiveness of the open learning materials once they are in regular use.

It is asserted that the potential of open learning can be realised in a range of scenarios, including Common Foundation/Branch Programmes, Enrolled Nurse Conversion Courses, and notably, in continuing education. Because of the interactive nature of the material, open learning unit extracts are excellent resources to use in institution-based sessions. They may need adapting to suit different sessions but they nevertheless provide good ideas for student-centred activities. Teachers may wish to use the following categories to judge the degree of openness of different materials and to assess their suitability for resource-based learning.

1.	Target group/users	multifarious . . . . . . specific
2.	Aims/objectives	broad . . . . . . specific
3.	Content	broad range . . . . . . narrow range
4.	Interactivity	group . . . . . . individual
5.	Learning methods/media	varied . . . . . . restricted
6.	Style	user friendly . . . . . . unfriendly
7.	Assessment	formative . . . . . . summative
8.	Impression	favourable . . . . . . unfavourable

It should be noted that the continua to the right of categories 1 to 7 do not necessarily imply a desirable . . . undesirable dimension, for example with reference to the first category, it may be considered very appropriate to address specific audiences such as senior education managers. To conclude this part of the chapter, teachers are asked to give further consideration to the potential of open/distance learning in their courses and how this mode of independent study may be fostered. Attention will now be focused on contract learning as an alternative mode of autarchic study.

Contract learning

A learning contract can be defined as a teaching/learning strategy where a student (or students) negotiates with his or her facilitator the objectives, methods for achieving the objectives, and criteria for evaluating his or her achievement of those objectives (Myles, 1990). Contracts can range from informal verbal to formal written agreements. Knowles (1984) identifies eight stages of a learning contract which can be condensed to five as follows:

(i)   assess learning needs with reference to a competency scale
(ii)   formulate appropriate objectives
(iii)   identify resources available with related actions and time frames
(iv)   carry out contract
(v)   evaluate learning outcomes against objectives of contract.

The five stages will now be discussed in more detail with reference to a worked example.

Stage 1   Learning needs – competency scale
Beattie's (1987) fourfold curriculum could be adapted for use as the basis for identifying a student's learning needs. In this example the student is in fact a teacher who wishes to develop his or her skills in the facilitation of independent study. To start with, Beattie's fourfold curriculum could be 'filled in' by the student teacher and his or her personal tutor conjointly, with the locus of control located with the student. The personal tutor acts as a facilitator using the data in Fig. 7.1 as a basis for the negotiation of learning needs.

Perceptive readers will have immediately spotted that the data in Fig. 7.1 is the essence of this chapter captured by Beattie's (1987) fourfold curriculum!

In our example the student teacher who wishes to develop his or her skills in facilitating independent study may decide to start with learning contracts. A competency scale as outlined in Fig. 7.2 could be used to identify his or her present knowledge ('P') and required ('R') knowledge base. It can be seen from the example in Fig. 7.2 that our student teacher has a degree of understanding of the nature and scope of learning contracts but wishes to use a contract to reduce the discrepancy between his or her preferred and required state. The value of using a competency scale (not a time-consuming exercise) is that it can be used to differentiate between different students' needs. Several students with different entry characteristics may wish to pursue the same area and the competency scales can help to personalise their learning contracts. However, some users may feel that the use of such a scale is redundant in a one-to-one relationship and an unnecessary prerequisite to the formulation of the learning objectives of the contract, but the author has found them useful.

Map of key subjects	Schedule of basic skills
open learning distance learning contract learning projects Keller plans (Personalised system of instruction) research	assess the suitability of open learning materials adapt open learning materials to suit local needs devise an acceptable framework for contract learning supervise project work/research
Portfolio of meaningful personal experiences	**Agenda of important cultural issues**
experiences with open learning research experience feelings about using learning contracts experience of computer assisted learning (CAL)	Project 2000 ENB/UKCC initiatives: future provision of continuing professional education

Fig. 7.1   Fourfold curriculum applied to independent study.

Knowledge of the principles and practice of learning contracts

Absent	Low		Moderate		High
	(awareness)		(understanding)		(expert)
0	1	2	3	4	5
		(P)		(R)	

Fig. 7.2   Competency scale.

Stage 2   Formulating appropriate learning objectives
The type of learning objectives used will depend on a range of factors
including:

- nature of the subject

- degree of discrepancy between 'P' and 'R' states

- relationship between contract and any formal scheme of assessment

- preferences of students/teachers

In our worked example the nature of the subject, i.e. learning contracts,

is primarily cognitive (and to some extent psychomotor) in nature. The discrepant relationship between the 'P' and 'R' suggests that our student teacher needs a more in-depth knowledge of the principles and practice of contract learning, particularly the role of the facilitator. It can be assumed that, in this example, our student can submit a written report on learning contracts as part of his or her formal scheme of assessment. It can also be assumed that both our student teacher and his or her personal tutor prefer general Tyler-type objectives and Eisner's express-ive outcomes as opposed to the highly specific and prescriptive format described by Mager (ENB, 1987).

Stage 3 Identify resources, actions needed, and time frames

This stage is best represented by considering how the learning contract for our student teacher might look. Figure 7.3 is a draft contract for our student teacher, based on a framework which has been adapted from Keyzer (1985). Several other frameworks exist (see ENB, 1989a) but users are encouraged to develop their own. Whatever framework is utilised, it is suggested that it is characterised by the following:

- simplicity
- user-friendliness
- actions and time frames
- locus of control with student
- adaptability

Stage 4 Carry out contract

During this stage the various actions agreed by the student teacher and his or her personal tutor are carried out with reference to the agreed time frames. During this phase of activity, aspects of the contract can be renegotiated by mutual consent. The role of the personal tutor would involve carrying out his or her part of the contract and offering other support, encouragement and guidance as appropriate. This reiterates the point made about extrinsic reinforcement earlier in the chapter.

Stage 5 Evaluate learning outcomes against objectives

During this stage the extent to which the 'P'—'R' discrepancy has been reduced is assessed. In other words, our student teacher is helped to assess whether he or she has achieved:

- none of the objectives
- some of the objectives
- all of the objectives
- different objectives
- all of the original plus different objectives

OBJECTIVES	RESOURCES	ACTIONS	TIME FRAMES	CRITERIA FOR EVALUATION
1. I wish to develop my knowledge of the principles and practice of learning contracts	1. Library 2. Librarian 3. Personal tutor	1. I will contact the librarian and undertake a literature search on learning contracts	3 days	1. I will produce a book and journal list which includes the most recent accounts on learning contracts
	As above	2. I will prepare a seminar paper for presentation to my peer group	10 days	2. I will present a seminar paper to my peer group which will include: (a) at least 3 definitions (b) the stages (c) at least 3 formats
	4. Peer group			3. I will facilitate a role-play with my peer group to experience negotiating a learning contract
				4. I will reassess my position on the competency scale using self-assessment and feedback from my peer group and personal tutor

Fig. 7.2 Sample learning contract for a student teacher

The answers to the above questions will influence what happens next. For example, our student teacher may renew his or her contract, negotiate a contract for another aspect of independent study, or negotiate an alternative form of learning experience.

In summary of this section, the use of learning contracts provides the opportunity for both teachers and students to individualise teaching and learning (Myles, 1990). However, it can be a time-consuming enterprise for all parties, especially for personal tutors. However, once students and their personal tutors are accustomed to their use, this can be less of a problem.

Attention will now be focused on projects as a mode of independent study.

Project methods/elective options

Good (1973) describes a project as 'a significant, practical unit of activity having educational value and aimed at one or more definite goals of understanding' (cited Adderley *et al.*, 1975). Curzon (1985) describes projects as part of the learning process, based on tasks carried out by students working individually or in groups and generally culminating in the presentation of a report. The term *student elective* is sometimes used to mean project work. Both Good's and Curzon's interpretations identify *student activity* and a *report* as the two main features of project work. Projects involve investigation and problem-solving, and frequently the use and manipulation of physical materials.

The education project is reported to have first appeared in America in 1908, denoting a specific unit of educational activity. It was used in connection with the courses in agriculture being run at the vocational schools in Massachusetts. The idea was that students of agriculture applied the material learned at school on the home farm or garden, thus performing a kind of empirical homework. Not all projects in higher education involve the manipulation of physical materials, but they commonly have the following characteristics.

1 They involve initiative by the student or group of students, and often necessitate a variety of educational activities.
2 They result in an end product, for example thesis, dissertation, report, dossier, design plans, computer programme, or learning package.
3 Work often goes on for a considerable length of time, though the time span may range from a single afternoon to three years or more.
4 The student is essentially autarchic, i.e. responsible for making his or her own decisions.

It is the fourth characteristic which qualifies projects as a mode of independent study as defined earlier in this chapter. Just as Dewey

(1916) advocated problem-solving approaches to education, Kilpatrick (1918) saw the project method as a tool for the student to control and direct his will through an educational experience which was morally defensible in a free society (cited Adderley *et al.*, 1975). Kilpatrick, the first to publish a systematic account and rationale of project methods, compared many traditional procedures in 'education' with the system of serfdom or slavery, where the individual's will was sublimated. Some elements of Dewey's and Kilpatrick's thinking are reflected in the ideologies of humanistic existentialism and andragogy which are currently popular with nurse educationalists.

Project work is further characterised by the following phases.

1 A briefing session during which the nature of the project is outlined, its aims clarified, and parameters determined.
2 A period of student investigation and design.
3 Presentation of the project.
4 Assessment and feedback.

The role of the personal tutor during each phase will now be explored. During phase 1, it may be necessary to have several tutorials with each student. Many students quickly decide on a theme whereas others need a longer period to decide on the nature and scope of their project. It is suggested that this phase is a shared venture between students and their supervisors, with the locus of control remaining with the students. Phase two represents the 'work up' period and is the most private part of the project. It is a period of 'incubation' and 'gestation' when the students gather and collate a mass of data. During this phase students often feel swamped and overwhelmed by the task. Personal tutors need to be sensitive to this situation arising, and be willing to provide support and guidance if sought. It is worth keeping a record of the project areas being pursued by each student to provide personal tutors with an appropriate mental set. Support and guidance tutorials can be most enriching experiences offering a great deal of job satisfaction. However, it must be stressed that the experiences can be time-consuming and exhausting if the tutor has a fairly large number of personal students.

During the presentation phase, personal tutors may suggest that students present their projects to each other. This can be accomplished through 'market stalls' where students can visit stalls which interest them. The final phase is characterised by assessment and feedback, an issue which has attracted much attention by different educationalists.

Assessment of projects/elective options

Warren Piper (1975) suggests that projects, perhaps more than any other method, raise problematic questions over assessment. This view is supported by Beard *et al.* (1978) who feel that the assessment of projects is particularly difficult. Hirst (1974) feels that it is essential that project assessors establish a well-defined list of criteria. Some internal examiners hold an oral examination, moderated by an external examiner, to clarify and expand on points covered in the project.

It is suggested that Warren Piper's and Beard's concerns regarding the assessment of project work relate to the problems of marking material of such a diverse nature. To illustrate this point, the following examples reflect the variety of elective options which may be submitted by student teachers as part of their assessment on a course with which the author is associated:

- an extended essay on an educational topic, e.g. adult learning

- a tape-slide programme, e.g. use of a nursing model in a practice area

- an academic game, e.g. a board game on wound healing

- an investigative study on teaching methods, e.g. contract learning

- a curriculum proposal, e.g. a Common Foundation Programme

- an open learning package, e.g. resources for health care assistants

- a health promotion video-cassette recording, e.g. low impact aerobics

On some secondary school courses in communication studies, students are required to prepare a project which requires a literature search, the classification and collation of data, and the preparation of a synopsis. The topics include organisational structure, radio programmes, and the processes involved in television broadcasts. This further reinforces the diversity of student projects and the problems of assessing such work. It is therefore proposed that teachers and students agree on a well-defined list of criteria which will be used to assess elective options. As mentioned previously, Hirst (1974) feels that it is essential to have clearly articulated criteria, but the author feels that the students should also 'own' the criteria if the spirit of andragogy is to be upheld.

Different criteria may be apposite for different kinds of project, for example a game versus open learning materials. However, the following could be used as 'core' criteria:

Presentation:	academic etiquette
	accuracy
	clarity
	synthesis
References:	comprehenive
	up-to-date
Originality:	inventive
	novel

Justification:	relevance
	worthwhileness
Educational:	evidence of evaluation
	underpinned by appropriate
	theory
Comprehensive:	breadth
	depth
Technical difficulty:	complex design
	use of technical resources

The use of an acronym, i.e. P-R-O-J-E-C-T, for the core criteria was intentional. The interpretation of those criteria merits further comment. Teachers and students should agree on the relative importance of each criterion since they do not necessarily carry equal weighting. For example, it could be argued that worthwhileness is of more importance than complexity of design. However, the criterion of worthwhileness is in itself value-laden. Teachers and students need to agree on what is meant by worthwhileness. In the case of a learning package, the potential benefit to the intended user group may serve as a 'yardstick' of worthwhileness. The involvement of external examiners in the negotiation of assessment criteria is also recommended since they often act for different centres which are likely to use different criteria.

Attention will now be focused on the relative merits of project work with reference to related literature and a small study conducted by the author.

Relative merits of project work as a mode of independent study

The student and qualified teachers with whom the author is involved are required to submit a project as part of their diploma or degree studies. A small study was carried out with 15 diploma students to assess the relative merits of project methods/elective options as claimed by Beard *et al.* (1978). Data was collected by personal interview with each student and a questionnaire. The findings will now be discussed under Beard, Bligh and Harding's categories.

1   Personal involvement   At its best, the project method is characterised by high levels of student activity, interest, enthusiasm, commitment and satisfaction. Fourteen students expressed enthusiasm and satisfaction from their efforts. The other student in the sample felt that the project was 'just another assignment' on the way to completing the course. She did concede that she had benefited from the exercise.

2 Skills for individual work All 15 students stated that they had gained much benefit from using their own initiative and resourcefulness. Seven students felt that their work would reap immediate dividends on return to their college of nursing. This was in fact later confirmed on a follow-up study day held for the students six months following course completion.

3 Skills for group work Nine students felt that they had been able to develop their ability to liaise with their colleagues in the practice setting. One good example of this was the production of a tape-slide programme for introducing a nursing model to a practice setting. This was well-received by the practice-based staff, who felt that the project had made a significant contribution to client-care.

4 Skills for communication Beard *et al.* (1978) suggest that project work affords students opportunities for practising communication skills through a variety of opportunities within the overall framework of the project. This claim can be supported with the following examples:

- teacher-student communication during all stages of the project

- student-student communication, especially with joint projects

- communication with nursing colleagues based in practice settings

- communication with relevant experts, e.g. statisticians in research projects.

Ten of the students in the study felt that their communication skills had developed through working on their electives.

5 Knowledge All 15 students stated that they had developed their skills at performing a literature search, and that they had become familiar with the methodology of their chosen subject areas. Three students reported a greater research awareness. Eleven students felt that they had achieved an in-depth knowledge of their subject area and that this had sustained their interest in their chosen specialism. All 15 students felt that working on their projects had helped them to integrate different subject areas, for example, nursing theory, educational psychology and curriculum studies.

6. Personal development Adderley *et al.* (1975) feel that a realistic assessment of one's own capabilities is essential for success in almost any profession. They feel that project work can leave students better equipped to face the challenges of professional life by helping them to realise their limitations and when and how to seek advice. The realisation of one's strengths and potential can be added to the debate, an advantage claimed by 11 of the 15 subjects in the sample.

The claimed disadvantages of project methods are as follows.

1   Teaching time   This can undoubtedly be a problem since each student may require at least one hour's tutorial. The contact time during the author's small study was three hours per student, some requiring more, and some requiring less.

2   Personality clashes   It is claimed that personality clashes between teachers and students can be an obstacle to progress. If this occurs, teachers and students should try and establish a more collegial relationship based on mutual trust and understanding.

3   Project work advantages the most able   It is suggested that project work affords the greatest advantage to the most able students. However, this was not found to be the case in the author's small study. Four of the students who had been performing satisfactorily in other areas (i.e. only average marks awarded for coursework) achieved a credit standard for their elective options. This was probably due to the fact that the subject areas were chosen by the students, reinforcing their personal commitment and motivation.

4   Assessment   The problems which surround the assessment of project work have been discussed. However, the author found that those students who had 'only' achieved a 'satisfactory' standard, were upset by the final grade (even though those students had performed at that level throughout the course). This was probably due to the personalised nature of project work and the amount of energy invested. This reinforces the assertion by Beard *et al.* that final grading may offset the advantages of feedback given at the conclusion of the project.

The limitations of such a small study are openly acknowledged and no generalisations are claimed. However, most of the advantages and disadvantages cited in the literature were upheld. It is asserted that the advantages of elective options outweigh the disadvantages provided that all attempts are made to improve the reliability and validity of assessment tools.

Summary

This chapter has attempted to analyse the concept of independent study with reference to the tenets of andragogy described by Knowles and the types of social need described by Bradshaw.

It was described as a predominantly autarchic mode of developing one's knowledge and skills, the locus of control resting with the student. However, the value of working in an interdependent manner was stressed. Different examples of working in an independent way were discussed. It could be argued that the different methods occupy different loci on a continuum of independence/interdependence as follows:

independence — — — — — — — — — — — — — — interdependence

| distance | open | contract | projects |
| learning | learning | learning | (joint) |

projects
(single)

Some open learning materials require that participants work in groups, shifting their locus to the right of the continuum. The nature and potential of open/distance learning were explored, particularly the steps which must be followed to ensure quality. A 'tool' for assessing the degree of 'openness' was outlined. A discussion on the stages of contract learning followed, suggesting how Beattie's fourfold curriculum could be used to identify learning needs with references to a competency scale. The design of 'user friendly' frameworks for learning contracts was recommended. The final example of independent study discussed in the main body of the chapter was that of projects/elective options. The nature, scope and relative merits of project methods were examined by comparing the findings in the literature with a small study conducted by the author. Particular attention was paid to the issues surrounding assessment, and the production of a list of core criteria to improve the reliability and validity of marking schemes was suggested.

Independent study is likely to claim its 'seat' on the 'front bench' of the 'party' of teaching/learning methods for some considerable time. Its 'policy' of self-determination is compatible with many prevailing ideologies in nursing education, notably humanism, humanistic existentialism, and andragogy. Open/distance learning is a cost-effective option when comparisons are made with institution-based courses. Contract learning affords students and their teachers the opportunity to individualise learning. Project methods encourage individual choice and commitment rather than ritualistic performance of set tasks. However, independent study should not be regarded as a 'cheap option' or 'cop out' by teachers since students may require considerable support during the process. Independent study is not regarded as the 'prime minister' of teaching/learning methods either. It is seen as an important component of a teacher's/student's 'tool-box' of strategies alongside other modes of learning.

References

Adderley, K.W. *et al.*   (1975).   *The Use of Project Methods in Higher Education.* Society for Research into Higher Education, London.

Beard, R.M. *et al.*   (1978).   *Research into Teaching Methods in Higher Education mainly in British Universities.* Fourth edition. Society for Research into Higher Education, London.

Beattie, A.   (1987).   Making a curriculum work. In *The Curriculum in Nursing Education*, P. Allan and M. Jolley (Eds), pp 15–34. Croom Helm, London.

Bernstein, B.   (1975).   *Class, Codes and Control – Vol. 3: Towards a Theory of Educational Transmissions.* Routledge and Kegan Paul, London.

Bradshaw, J.   (1972).   The concept of social need. *New Society*, **No. 496**, 640–3.

Chin, R. and Benne, K.D.   (1985).   General strategies for effecting change in human systems. In *Planning of Change.* Fourth edition. W.G. Bennis *et al.* (Eds), pp 22–45. Holt, Rinehart and Winston, New York.

Collins Pocket Dictionary of the English Language   (1981).   Collins, London.

Curzon, L.B.   (1985). *Teaching in Further Education.* Third Edition. Holt, Rinehart and Winston, London.

English National Board for Nursing, Midwifery and Health Visiting   (1987).   *Managing Change in Nursing Education – Section 1: Preparing for Change.* ENB, London.

English National Board for Nursing, Midwifery and Health Visiting   (1989a). *Managing Change in Nursing Education – Section 2: Workshop Materials for Action.* ENB, London.

English National Board for Nursing, Midwifery and Health Visiting   (1989b).   *Project 2000 – 'A New Preparation for Practice': Guidelines and Criteria for Course Development and the Formation of Collaborative Links Between Approved Training Institutions Within the National Health Service and Centres of Higher Education.* ENB, London.

Hirst, P.H.   (1974).   *Knowledge and the Curriculum.* Routledge and Kegan Paul, London.

Holland, S.   (1989).   Open learning: ensuring quality. *Nursing Standard*, **4(1)**, 26–9.

Jarvis, P.   (1983).   *Adult and Continuing Education: Theory and Practice.* Croom Helm, London.

Keyzer, D.M.   (1985).   *Learning Contracts, the Trained Nurse and the Implementation of the Nursing Process.* Ph.D. thesis. Institute of Education, University of London, London.

Knowles, M.S.   (1984).   *Andragogy in Action.* Jossey Bass, San Francisco.

Mezirow, J.   (1981).   A critical theory of adult learning and education. In *Adult Learning and Education*, M. Tight (Ed.), pp 5–13. Croom Helm, London.

Myles, A.P.   (1990).   Curriculum pathways to Project 2000. In *Nursing: a Knowledge Base for Practice*, A. Perry and M. Jolley (Eds). Edward Arnold, Sevenoaks.

Quinn, F.M.   (1988).   *The Principles and Practice of Nurse Education.* Second edition. Croom Helm, London.

8 Evaluating teaching effectiveness

Valerie Lattimer

If you are a teacher, ask yourself a question: do you consider yourself to be an average, above average or below average teacher? Cross (1977) asked teachers this question and reported that an 'amazing' 94% of his sample rated themselves as above average teachers; 68% estimated that they would be in the top quarter in terms of teaching performance (cited by Ericksen, 1985). These remarkable results may not in themselves be significant, but they raise questions about the information on which the teachers in the Cross sample made their estimation. On what information was your self-rating based? How important is it that nurse teachers are able to account for their effectiveness?

The United Kingdom Central Council for Nursing, Midwifery and Health Visiting advisory document *Exercising Accountability* (UKCC, 1989) reiterates that each registered nurse, midwife, and health visitor is accountable for his or her practice, and, in its summary of principles, advises that 'The exercise of accountability requires the practitioner to seek to achieve and to maintain high standards.' By definition, nurse teachers share this accountability for practice. Written standards for practice in nurse education may encapsulate the notion of 'good teaching' while the development of performance indicators and performance review are enabling nurse educators to explore ways of improving the quality of nurse teaching. Of significance for the nurse teacher is the need to maintain high standards of practice and to continue to develop and respond to change. How, on a day to day basis, can nurse teachers evaluate their effectiveness? This chapter seeks to address this question. First, however, it is necessary to clarify what is meant by the terms 'good teaching', 'effectiveness', and 'evaluation'.

A broad statement about *teaching* is needed if it is to encompass the personal perceptions of teachers about the activities of teaching; to define teaching may be to limit its potentiality. According to Braskamp *et al.* (1984), teaching is 'related to student learning and deals with establishing conditions for facilitating learning.' A helpful starting point for teachers who wish to reflect upon their practice is to identify their own beliefs about teaching and its aims. Some educators question the relationship between teaching and learning, for example Braskamp *et al.* (1984) prefer to describe it as a 'possible' relationship while Delamont (1984) asserts that there is no clear evidence that good teachers maximise pupil learning. Clearly the many variables which affect learning make it difficult to isolate precisely the effects of teaching upon learning. For this reason, only using assessment of student learning as a measure of effective teaching is not recommended. Given these difficulties, evaluating teaching may appear too difficult a task but Ericksen (1985) emphasises that 'good teaching is not something which can be taken for granted ... evaluative checks and balances will always be needed to guard the welfare of students, individual teachers and the institutions.' For Van Ort *et al.* (1986), evaluating teaching is more than an important component of curriculum evaluation: 'It reflects the mission and goals of the institution, the goals and expectations of its programs and the level of education, preparation and experience of the faculty.' Gallego (1987) warns that if nurse teaching is to survive it needs to develop evaluation models which illuminate both its worth and cost effectiveness.

Applegate (1981) proposes five alternative models for documenting *teaching effectiveness*; the models could be used in combination. These include a criterion-based model where teachers' performance is measured against set standards; a development model for teacher growth and development; and a personnel decision-making model (cited by Van Ort *et al.*, 1986). A distinction needs to be made here between evaluating teaching for the purpose of teacher self-improvement and evaluating teaching for the purpose of informing personnel decision-making. How evaluation information will be used is critical; the purpose of teacher evaluation must be known and evaluation results used only for the purpose identified. Difficulties could be foreseen, for example, if the results of a diagnostic classroom teaching evaluation intended purely for self-development were used as evidence at performance review. This is not to be pedantic but rather to emphasise that information collected about the performance of persons is sensitive. Even though Braskamp *et al.* (1984) suggest that with careful planning the needs of both the organisation and the teacher can be met within the same evaluation exercise, they stress that this can be difficult to achieve. If it can be agreed that evaluative checks and balances are needed in nurse education despite the complexity of teaching, then perhaps it is reasonable to suggest that a *complete* evaluation of teaching is neither possible nor necessary. As Seibert (1979) maintains, 'the arts of effective teaching are too numerous, varied and subtle to be accounted for fully, much less simply' (cited by Ericksen, 1985). It is necessary, therefore, to consider what aspects of nurse teaching ought to be evaluated and how this evaluation might be achieved.

Beeby (1975) defines *evaluation* as 'the systematic collection and interpretation of evidence, leading, as part of the process to a judgement of value with a view of action (cited by Wolf, 1979). Key issues are highlighted in this definition and are worthy of further discussion.

Some key issues in evaluation

The systematic collection of evidence

Does evaluation differ from research? This question underpins much of the debate within the field of general education, a debate which has intensified over the last twenty years. Principally, the quantitative versus qualitative debate is alive and well here but can involve the novice evaluator in some intellectual acrobatics in an attempt to get it right. At the risk of over simplifying the debate the central issues will be pursued here.

Adelman and Alexander (1987) contentiously describe the debate as 'the dichotomy between pure research versus impure evaluation, the objective versus the subjective and the scientific versus the unscientific.' For Wolf (1979), research aims to produce new and generalisable knowledge which may have no specific reference to any practical dimension, while evaluation is deliberately undertaken as a guide to action. Hence the strength of experimental research is that it may enable generalisations to be made, but its chief weakness is that it may ignore the more subtle events of teaching and learning. Classroom research, then, is not synonymous with teacher evaluation. The view of Murphy and Torrance (1987) is that the 'tradition in education has been one of asserting the importance of qualitative understandings of educational processes over the quantitative measurement of the outcomes of such processes.' In an attempt to encourage clarity, Stenhouse (1987) recommends the use of the word 'evidence' as opposed to 'data' when describing the results of evaluative work. In defence of evaluative work, Wolf (1979) asserts that evaluation and research are not the same and that 'the methodologies of the latter do not need to dictate the activities of the former.' For the purpose of evaluating the effectiveness of teaching, generalisability of findings is not aspired to, although teachers who share their experiences of evaluating may identify some common areas for discussion. Delamont (1984) reflects that, in the past in general education, much classroom description has been behavioural and that 'classroom research cannot afford to divorce what people do from their intentions.' Qualitative or illuminative work in the evaluation of teaching seeks to examine the processes as well as the products of education. Of illuminative evaluation in an educational setting Parlett and Hamilton (1987) state that the chief task is to unravel the complex scene, 'isolate its significant features; delineate cycles of cause and effect; and comprehend relationships between beliefs and practices, and between organizational patterns and the responses of individuals.'

Parlett and Hamilton (1987) further assert that the primary concern of illuminative evaluation is with 'description and interpretation rather than measurement and prediction.' To return to Beeby's (1975) definition (cited by Wolf, 1979) this need not mean, however, that such evaluation utilises unsystematic techniques.

Making judgements of value with a view to action

The action component of evaluation is seen by some writers to be necessary to justify the resources required by the process. In other words, evaluating for its own sake is not worthwhile. Cronbach (1987) regards evaluation as 'the collection and use of information to make decisions about an educational programme.' Information arising out of evaluation for self-improvement would contribute to a reflection on, and possibly change in, practice. Making judgements of value poses a rather more difficult problem. While Flanders (1970) acknowledges that 'it seems almost impossible to study classroom interaction without developing value judgements about what is going on and beginning to imagine alternatives', making value judgements is essentially a subjective activity and as such is the focus of criticism for the quantitative researcher. Parlett and Hamilton (1987) would argue that the external illuminative evaluator should endeavour to expose subjective elements of the evaluation and acknowledge them. For example at the report stage, 'in addition to the findings, critical research processes can also be documented: theoretical principles and methodological ground rules can be discussed and made explicit; criteria for selecting or rejecting areas of investigation can be spelled out; and evidence can be presented in such a way that others can judge its quality'. Making value judgements is part of the evaluation process, but in this way the subjective element is acknowledged and openly discussed and, in itself, may prove to be illuminative. The evaluation of nurse teaching might be enriched by adopting the principles of illuminative evaluation, and novice evaluators can take heart from Stronach's (1987) comment that there 'are experts *about* evaluation, but not expert evaluators.' It is a difficult task to find a workable compromise between quantitative and qualitative approaches, yet to ignore the debate is to fail to learn from the wealth of educational studies of the past. Perhaps the starting point for nurse teachers is to have the confidence to make a start, for as Gallego (1987) urges 'the important aspect is to break new ground and plant the seed'.

Making a start: needs and problems for the nurse teacher

Gallego (1983) asserts that 'evaluation in nursing education lags behind developments in general education'. A recent literature review appears to confirm this observation. This is not to suggest that evaluation is not undertaken by nurse teachers. Some evaluation of teaching is essential for courses to be run and course evaluation may include obtaining student evaluation of teaching. Teachers frequently respond to the needs of students by altering timetables, having a flexible lesson plan and so on. Rather, the evaluation of teaching as opposed to the evaluation of courses could benefit from a more informed and planned approach. A system of evaluating can offer the teacher a useful framework and may encourage the evaluation of aspects of teacher practice which the teacher might not otherwise choose to examine.

It would seem that the next step is to explore the range of evaluation techniques available, make appropriate selections and encourage their use. However, it is important first to try and establish the particular needs of the nurse teacher in this respect.

Most evaluation of teaching in general education is concerned with classroom-centred work. Nurse teachers work in other settings, the clinical setting for example and, like teachers in general education, operate in roles other than teacher during their work: mentor to unqualified teachers, member of a working party, personal tutor to students and so on. Nurse teachers need a model for evaluating practice which has relevance for these aspects of the role. Traditionally evaluation of teaching has used the locus of the classroom. There are no evaluation systems designed specifically for the nurse teacher which take account of other dimensions of the role. Any classroom evaluation therefore, however methodologically rigorous, on its own fails to account fully for the work of the nurse teacher. If methods which enable 'knowing' about effectiveness can only provide an incomplete picture, then perhaps nurse teachers have been more willing to be satisfied with their 'feelings' about effectiveness. While acknowledging that each educational establishment in which nurse teachers work has its own staff structure, a common system of working appears to be that of the team.

In the author's experience the realities of working as a member of a teaching team are sometimes at a tangent to the ideology of team work. All too often individual teachers can become isolated as they accept and develop responsibility for courses, groups of learners, or specialist aspects of teaching. For some this may be a preferred way of working, for others, in particular unqualified or newly qualified teachers, this can be a difficult experience. The feeling of being part of a team can be lost even though the structure and mechanics of team management remain. This is not necessarily a reflection on the management style of the team leader, rather a reminder that a team is not necessarily a group. A group, defined by Zander (1982) is 'a collection or set of individuals who interact with and depend on each other'. A body of people is *not* a group 'if the members are primarily interested in individual accomplishments, are not concerned with the activities of other members or see others as rivals, and are often absent from meetings'. The assignment of tasks to individuals within teams can lead to the assignment of total responsibility for those tasks, and though the effective teacher may enjoy the success experience of being effective and being known to be effective this may be at the cost of some considerable stress in juggling priorities alone. Of course team members do help each other and may have effective working relationships, but nevertheless there is the propensity for team working to lead to negative experiences for the teacher.

Whether or not teachers work in teams they are constrained by the demands of the organisation. A nurse teacher is essentially a post holder, carrying out the role as defined by the organisation. Although roles do develop, Ericksen (1985) observes that 'it takes courage to march to a different beat than the one given by the Dean or the power structure within the department'. It does, however, depend upon how strong the beat is. Any cross sectional study of nurse teachers working to the same job description is likely to reveal that each teacher perceives his or her role differently and executes it accordingly. Some aspects of the role will be seen to be more important than others; these will probably not be the same aspects. Organisations can generally tolerate this variance, indeed it can be seen to enrich the provision that the organisation can make. It may be significant, however, when evaluating teacher effectiveness to ask to what extent teacher behaviour is influenced by the demands made by the organisation. Performance review may already be making a significant contribution to teacher evaluation but its aims are subtly different. It is essentially used to obtain evidence that the employee is fulfilling the role required of him or her by the organisation. This is not to deny that performance review can contribute to teacher development and that, in itself, it is a useful exercise, but to observe that the decision to initiate performance review is made by the manager, not the teacher. Hence even the formative aspects of performance review may be perceived as summative.

Evaluation strategies

It is likely that no one evaluation strategy alone can fully illuminate the work of the nurse teacher. The presence of a subjective element in evaluation has been established and for this reason the use of a combination of evaluation techniques is recommended. In this way some degree of triangulation might be achieved which would strengthen the evaluation evidence. In broad terms, inclusion of self, peer, and student evaluation is desirable. A selection of helpful evaluation strategies will be proposed for each dimension, although the reader will find others in the literature.

Self-evaluation

The author's experience as mentor to student teachers is that their enthusiasm is accompanied by a willingness to be open, to take risks and to reflect on experience. Reflecting on the experience of teaching is central to self-evaluation. It requires the teachers to be alive and responsive to the group, and to be conscious of themselves during the process. After the event the teacher needs time to reflect, time which may be difficult to make space for in a busy schedule. Hence, qualified nurse teachers may lose the opportunity rather than the ability for self-evaluation. Braskamp *et al.* (1984) regard self-evaluation of teaching as 'a necessary condition for change and growth'. Teachers may be required to submit a written self-evaluation as part of performance review, but for the purpose of less formal evaluation there are other alternatives. English National Board for Nursing, Midwifery and Health Visiting (1987) contains a valuable section entitled 'Assessing your own approach' (section 1.3) which enables the nurse teacher to make a detailed assessment of overall teaching style and performance. From a state of awareness of one's teaching preferences and behaviour it is possible to work towards identified goals for change. The self-evaluation of smaller identifiable units of teaching can be achieved in a loosely structured way by taking time out, preferably soon after the event to ask oneself broad questions such as:

* What went well?
* What would I change if I were to repeat this, and why? Or more specific questions such as:
* Were my aims achieved? Were they realistic?
* Did I make best use of the available resources?

The reality of nurse teachers having this sort of conversation with themselves may appear unlikely, yet it is a simple, viable, and pragmatic strategy which has application for the range of the nurse teachers' activities. For many teachers this self-evaluation is a feature of their work, even if time is not deliberately set aside for it. Combining self-evaluation with student or peer-evaluation can minimise the subjectivity which is the main criticism of this technique.

Evaluation by students

Seeking student opinion about educational programmes is generally accepted practice in nurse education. Means of collecting this information may vary from writing on blank sheets of paper to completing more structured questionnaires; from teacher led group discussions to student-centred personal interviews. Students are undoubtedly in a unique position to offer feedback to teachers as they are the focus of the teacher's activity, or, in the words of Ericksen (1985), 'have ringside seats'; but there are both advantages and limitations involved with the use of student evaluations. Ericksen (1985) reports that the combined observations of students provide a 'degree of consistency that cannot be matched by a single opinion' and Seibert (1979) states that reliability of student ratings is particularly good where pre-tested question items are used (cited by Ericksen, 1985). These can enable the teacher to evaluate specific aspects of a course or session. Where students are not helped to give feedback there is a risk that entertainment value becomes tied too closely to educational value. Braskamp *et al.* (1984) suggest that students are better at writing what they liked or disliked, or considered to be worthwhile or worthless, than analysing why or making suggestions for improving the course structure or teaching style. On the extent to which student judgements are related to good teaching, Ericksen points out that 'students may know some things about their teachers but not everything'. It is important, according to Wood and Matthewman (1987), that evaluations are not based on factors which are beyond the teacher's control, particularly as variables such as the size of the class and whether or not the course is compulsory are known to affect student ratings. Braskamp *et al.* (1984) warn against the 'over-kill' which can result from too frequent evaluation.

The question of whether students should sign written responses is controversial, and while Braskamp *et al.* (1984) recommend that they are not asked to do so, Ericksen (1985) maintains that 'unsigned criticism has little to do with accountability and violates the rights of the teacher as an academic citizen'. With regard to the destiny of written comments, it is important that this should be known to the students. Comments may, for example, be seen by senior teachers and guest speakers and this should be made clear to students. The timing of written evaluation is another key issue. The 'Friday afternoon evaluation', for instance, may be a rushed affair and fail to provide information about the longer term worthwhileness of an educational programme. Furthermore, while the image of students having ringside seats is an engaging one, it rather lends itself to an impression that teaching is something which happens to students rather than something with which they are intrinsically involved. In relation to this, the practice of asking students to evaluate their own contributions to a session has much to commend it. With regard to the mode of obtaining feedback from students it could be argued that by using written evaluations alone an opportunity to develop their skills of verbal feedback is missed. The Nominal Group Technique is an example of the qualitative tool which combines both written and verbal techniques and which, in the author's experience, proved to be illuminative and flexible enough for use in the clinical and classroom setting. A quantitative element can be included if desired.

The Nominal Group Technique (Delbecq *et al.*, 1975)

This technique has essentially five stages:

- The person conducting the session identifies key questions. These are open questions which aim to facilitate a breadth of response, for example:
  What were the strengths of the series of sessions?
  How could the sessions have been improved?
Questions can be used as headings on flip chart paper for example.

- Individuals write down their own ideas.

- Participants form groups then collate their ideas on paper, each person in turn adding an idea until the group feel that there is nothing more to add. There is no discussion at this stage.

- The group then discuss the ideas in order to clarify meanings and to combine contributions which are similar.

- A large group discussion follows. Participants may elect to vote in private for items they feel strongly about, hence the teacher can come to know which items have the strongest support of the group.

An important strength of the technique is that the students' own words are used and are not amended by the teacher, thus retaining original meanings. Focusing on strengths and improvements creates balance. This technique could also be used to evaluate a clinical experience, or an entire course by adapting the key questions. While Braskamp *et al.* (1984) have some reservations about the ability of students to suggest course or teacher improvements, in the author's experience this technique can facilitate pertinent and thoughtful suggestions by students. By seeking out the opinions of students, and by planning to set aside some considerable time to do so, the teacher implicitly values them. The technique has the strengths of a questionnaire in that every student makes a comment but without the pre-set agenda of a questionnaire which can tend to focus on what the teacher wants to know rather than what the student wants to say. The technique has the strengths of a group discussion without the disadvantages of a large group experience where some individuals may feel unable to contribute. The technique does have one limitation; a minimum of two hours is required to complete the process. The brainstorming and voting phases can be followed by feedback and discussion with the teacher at a later time if this is more convenient, although delay may diminish the ability of students to remember precisely what was meant by the written comments.

Alternative tools for evaluating the effectiveness of nurse teaching in the clinical setting are plentiful in literature from the USA (Mogan and Knox, 1987; Pacini and Westphal, 1988; Wood and Matthewman, 1987; Zimmerman and Westfall, 1988). A favoured framework appears to be the rating scale questionnaire. Preliminary work on these tools aimed to identify effective behaviour of clinical teachers. From this, statements of effective behaviour were written and form the basis of student evaluation. Zimmerman and Westfall (1988) list 43 such statements, for example: 'Identifies principles basic to practice; assists students in understanding their professional responsibility; corrects students tactfully; stimulates students to think about using research to improve patient care'. In the United Kingdom, the clinical teacher to student ratio is likely to limit the use of this type of tool. In order to be able to respond to the items the student would need to have spent more considerable time with the clinical teacher. It is important, however, that, for nurse teachers in the clinical settings, the opportunity to evaluate their practice is not overlooked because of methodological difficulty alone.

Evaluation by peers

In peer review the teacher obtains the co-operation of a colleague or colleagues. It is desirable for the teacher to select a colleague with whom she or he feels comfortable or who she or he thinks has particular skills to offer. For some teachers, the notion of evaluating teaching in any other way than by self-appraisal will be controversial. It represents a direct exposure of the self to others. Flanders (1970) writes about the need to avoid enquiry into teacher effectiveness becoming 'an intellectual, emotional and spiritual striptease'. 'Personal illusions need not be peeled off one by one.' Instead 'a constructive enquiry into existing behaviour and alternatives for change can be planned and carried out.' Ericksen (1985) agrees that 'in the absence of trust, any evaluation scheme is doomed to flounder'. Ewan and White (1984) make an obvious but important point when they suggest that 'an approach which stresses mutual co-operation among teachers will be more helpful than one in which teachers are encouraged to criticize each other's efforts'. Peer review may overcome some of the potential shortcomings of self-evaluation used alone. One obstacle to self-evaluation is what Flanders (1970) describes as 'the personal illusions which often confound improvement'. Peer review provides an opportunity to confront personal illusions and can help those teachers who find it difficult to identify for themselves the positive aspects of their teaching.

Cohen and McKeachie (1980) suggest that peers are able to evaluate some aspects of the teacher's work particularly well. These include:
- Depth and breadth of knowledge related to what is being taught
- Selection of course content and its organisation
- Appropriate use of resource materials – readings and audio-visual media, for example

- Quality of student assessment – tests, papers, and projects
- Teaching methods consistent with course substance
- Commitment to teaching, to students, and to the instructional program of the department.

(cited by Ericksen, 1985).

The use of peers in the evaluation of the process of teaching is particularly helpful. Unless audiovisual recordings of teaching are made the teacher has difficulty in reviewing the process alone. A major contribution to the study of the process of teaching has been made by the interaction analysis school which uses systematic, non-participant observation to collect evidence about teacher behaviour. One of the best known systems, and an example of a quantitative approach to teacher evaluation, is that of Flanders (1970). The basis of interaction analysis in the classroom context is explained as follows by Flanders: 'teaching behaviour by its very nature exists in a context of social interaction. The acts of teaching lead to reciprocal contacts between the teacher and the pupils, and the interchange itself is called teaching. Techniques for analyzing classroom interaction are based on the notion that these reciprocal contacts can be perceived as a series of events which occur one after another.' In Flanders' terms an event is 'the shortest possible act that a trained observer can identify and record.'

Flanders sorted teaching behaviour into ten categories (Fig. 8.1). Seven of these categories relate to teacher talk and two to pupil talk, with one category for silence or confusion. A trained observer uses a time schedule in conjunction with the categories to record the behaviour of the teacher at approximately three second intervals. A profile of classroom interaction emerges. Interaction analysis in itself does not make value judgements about which categories are effective, rather it facilitates a sorting out of complex events. It may be illuminative for teachers to be aware of which categories they use most. In support of the system Croll (1986), argues that, while it is an extremely simple system, 'a combination of the continuing relevance of the distinctions made by the categories with an extremely sophisticated approach to data analysis has meant that the system can provide a wealth of information about teaching processes.' Training for observers is required; Flanders (1970) proposed that between four and twelve hours of practice and recording would be sufficient to safeguard inter-observer reliability. For nurse teachers who are not planning to use the interaction analysis categories to undertake classroom research this requirement is not as important, particularly where it is being used to provide formative feedback.

Interaction analysis has however been the focus of some criticism. Systematic observation is concerned with observable behaviour and critics of this technique argue that subtle but possibly important events could be missed. Delamont (1984) warns that 'to the extent that classroom research claims to illuminate the processes associated with class-

Teacher Talk	Response	1. *Accepts feeling.* Accepts and clarifies an attitude or the feeling tone of a pupil in a non-threatening manner. Feelings may be positive or negative. Predicting and recalling feelings are included. 2. *Praises or encourages.* Praises or encourages pupil action or behavior. Jokes that release tension, but not at the expense of another individual; nodding head, or saying 'Um hm?' or 'go on' are included. 3. *Accepts or uses ideas of pupils.* Clarifying, building, or developing ideas suggested by a pupil. Teacher extensions of pupil ideas are included but as the teacher brings more of his own ideas into play, shift to category five.
		4. *Asks questions.* Asking a question about content or procedure, based on teacher ideas, with the intent that a pupil will answer.
	Initiation	5. *Lecturing.* Giving facts or opinions about content or procedures; expressing *his own* ideas, giving *his own* explanation, or citing an authority other than a pupil. 6. *Giving directions.* Directions, commands, or orders to which a pupil is expected to comply. 7. *Criticizing or justifying authority.* Statements intended to change pupil behavior from non-acceptable to acceptable pattern; bawling someone out; stating why the teacher is doing what he is doing; extreme self-reference.
Pupil Talk	Response	8. *Pupil-talk – response.* Talk by pupils in response to teacher. Teacher initiates the contact or solicits pupil statement or structures the situation. Freedom to express own ideas is limited.
	Initiation	9. *Pupil-talk – initiation.* Talk by pupils which they initiate. Expressing own ideas; initiating a new topic; freedom to develop opinions and a line of thought, like asking thoughtful questions; going beyond the existing structure.
Silence		10. *Silence or confusion.* Pauses, short periods of silence and periods of confusion in which communication cannot be understood by the observer.

Fig. 8.1 Flanders' (1970) Interaction Analysis Categories (FIAC).* There is *no* scale implied by these numbers. Each number is classifactory; it designates a particular kind of communication event. To write these numbers down during observation is to enumerate, not to judge a position on a scale.

room life, it cannot afford to divorce what people do from their intentions.' In his writing, Flanders appears to acknowledge this when he advises that 'a more flexible technique is required when more subtle distinctions are necessary.' Clearly the quality of recording will depend in part on the skill of the observer, and the presence of an observer in the classroom will have some effect on interaction. However, the effects may not be as great if the observer is another teacher known to the students. Supporters of the illuminative approach to evaluation might argue that providing the observer effect is acknowledged it need not affect the quality of the evidence. While Ericksen (1985) asserts that in the final analysis the concepts which students come to understand are more important than the teaching style they observe, Eble (1980) maintains that 'teaching style is not a superficial but a consistent display of the real character and values of the teacher' (cited by Ericksen, 1985).

As a tool for diagnostic work, systematic observation has good potential. For example, if a videotape recording of a session is made, this enables the teacher to analyse her or his own behaviour with the important additional insight of knowing what was intended. Croll (1986) is enthusiastic about the use of videotape in this way and Delamont (1984) reflects that the 'use of interaction analysis in this way brings it much closer to the ethnographic research model.'

Guidelines for using audiotape and audiovisual feedback

Watching self on videotape can be perturbing. One can be equally absorbed and mortified by a display of mannerisms and behaviour that is barely recognised as self. In recognising this tendency Croll (1986) recommends viewing the videotape in conjunction with the interaction analysis categories in order that the teacher is helped to look beyond the behaviour. Walker (1987) is interested in developing the natural observational skills of teachers and cites the work of Ireland and Russell (1978) who developed a method called 'pattern analysis' using audiotape. In pattern analysis a session is audiotaped and then a small portion of the tape (approximately five minutes in length) is transcribed word for word. Subsequent reading through the transcript enables the teacher to identify recurring patterns or forms of interaction which are then described as objectively as possible. Audio and audiovisual recordings cannot recreate the real experience and in this sense will always be deficient, but unlike reality they can be revisited again and again. Moreover, citing the work of Chapman (1978), Jeffers and Guthrie (1988) recall that 'individuals who use videotaping as a means to self-evaluate identified decreased levels of teaching anxiety, increased levels of self-confidence, and enhanced attention to specific behaviours important to teaching others.' This would suggest that the transition to the action stage of evaluation was effective in this example. Sharing the review of the recordings with a colleague as a method of peer review may help the teacher to explore alternatives and importantly 'to work through some of the personal reactions to evaluations, especially the negative ones' (Braskamp *et al.*, 1984).

Improving evaluation in nurse education: Cluster centred practice

Given the range of evaluation strategies available to the nurse teacher, it could be assumed that making teachers aware of them is to have done enough. These strategies are not new; they have been available from educational literature for some time. Many teachers will be familiar with some of, if not all, the techniques. However, there is danger that the simplest option, a 'tacked on to existing practice' approach would be ineffective because it fails to deal with the constraints facing nurse teachers, or to examine why evaluation strategies might be under-developed. For the evaluation of teacher effectiveness to be more than a 'good idea', perhaps what is required is a change in the way in which nurse teachers work.

Lattimer and Lattimer (1989) propose 'cluster centred practice' as a potential development of the work of the nurse teacher. The central concept in this proposal is the 'cluster'. A cluster is a group of three practitioners (in this case teachers) who work together and also have shared responsibility for work. The term 'cluster' is important because while it suggests a closeness of relationship between members it does not prescribe their roles. In particular there is no organisationally identified leader, rather each cluster member will lead from time to time. A three member cluster is proposed as it generates optimum opportunity for communicating and sharing without the difficulties of reaching consensus which can be a feature of larger groups. The evidence from Sampson and Marthas (1977) is that 'a dyad permits a relationship with only one other, a triad six relationships (the six combinations of the three persons). A group of four persons allows twenty five possible relationships.'

Clusters would ideally be self-selected but would be guided by the needs of the organisation. For example, the curriculum may demand the formation of specialist rather than generalist clusters with respect to teacher expertise. Ultimately the organisation retains the right to select clusters and as such retains its overriding authority. If a teacher was seen by others in the cluster to be 'difficult', working through this could be part of the professional development of the group; although as Zander (1982) points out, 'persons whose beliefs do not fit together well have a hard time forming a strong group.' A senior teacher would effectively be a consultant to several clusters and would retain line management responsibility. Clusters, although close groups, are not closed groups.

Clusters in practice

Clusters could be a viable working strategy for teachers who are based in the clinical setting. The isolation which can be experienced by clinically based nurse teachers would at least be addressed. As many nurse teachers prepare for a different clinical role, this could be a unique opportunity to share and learn from the experience of colleagues. Clusters would plan work together. This could enable a more even and sustained level of work than the present team oriented system provides for individual teachers, in which there can be peaks and troughs of demand. Priority setting would reflect the work of the cluster and time-limited work could be effected more quickly. There is likely to be a tendency for the group to develop its own motivation to meet agreed objectives or indeed to assert that more time or resources are needed. Mann and Likert (1977) observed that 'Group pressure can reinforce reciprocal expectations for members to carry out decisions agreed to by the group.' Clearly individuals will continue to implement aspects of work alone but being part of a cluster will mean that at least two other individuals will have identified themselves as essential resources. Communication between senior teachers and individual teachers would continue but the whole cluster would need to be involved in discussions about its work. Meetings with the other clusters supervised by the senior teacher would be important to facilitate the exchange of information and ideas and for maintaining contact between clusters.

A potential problem with clusters is that they could fall victim to 'group think' and become mutually exclusive. Providing that links between clusters can be maintained this problem should be avoided. In any case clusters are likely to develop links with each other where resources are shared or mutual co-operation is advantageous. The informal and highly developed colleague network which would pre-date a cluster arrangement would of course continue. With particular reference to Project 2000 courses, a cluster system could enable teaching colleagues or specialists from other departments to link in with a group. This may increase the likelihood that visiting teachers will feel comfortable and have a sense of belonging.

Integration of teaching can readily be discussed, hence the risk that links may not be made to other course content is more likely to be avoided. For inexperienced teachers or student teachers on teaching practice, a cluster could offer an educationally orientated and personally supportive milieu. This could make a significant contribution to the prevention of the experience of marginality which occurs when an individual takes on a role within an institution which is peripheral to the main functioning of that institution (Burns, 1982).

Clusters and the evaluation of teaching effectiveness

There are several ways in which cluster centred practice might facilitate teacher evaluation.

- The evaluation of the teaching effectiveness of individuals has a forum and the human resources it requires.

- This forum will enable the discussion of action plans, together with support for teachers implementing such plans.

- Mutual support is more likely to facilitate the risk taking which is a feature of trying out new approaches.

- From closer working relationships and shared responsibility, trust is more likely to develop. Trust is necessary for sharing and peer review.

- Working together, sharing ideas and resources, challenging existing practice all would help to generate the enthusiasm and energy which is a prerequisite for change.

This chapter has addressed the need for nurse teachers to develop the evaluation of their effectiveness. A selection of approaches has been reviewed which might contribute to this development, including cluster centred practice. While it clearly remains to be seen whether this proposal could succeed, it may not be too remote from existing practice to warrant further investigation.

References

Adelman, C. and Alexander, R. (1987). The integrity of evaluation. In *Evaluating Education: Issues and Methods*, R. Murphy and H. Torrance (Eds), pp 294–310. Harper and Row, London.

Braskamp, L.A. *et al.* (1984). *Evaluating Teaching Effectiveness*. Sage, Beverley Hills.

Burns, R. (1982). *Self-Concept Development and Education*. Holt, Rinehart and Winston, London.

Croll, P. (1986). *Systematic Classroom Observation*. Falmer Press, London.

Cronbach, L. (1987). Issues in planning evaluations. In *Evaluating Education: Issues and Methods*, R. Murphy and H. Torrance (Eds), pp 4–35. Harper and Row, London.

Delamont, S. (1984). Revisiting classroom research: a cautionary tale. In *Readings on Interaction in the Classroom*, S. Delamont (Ed.), pp. 3–24. Methuen, London.

Delbecq, A. *et al.* (1975). *Group Techniques for Program Planning: A Guide to Nominal Group and Delphi Processes*. Scott, Foresman & Co., Glenview, Illinois.

English National Board for Nursing, Midwifery and Health
Visiting (1987). *Managing Change in Nursing Education – Section 1:
Preparing For Change*. ENB, London.

Ericksen, S.C. (1985). *The Essence of Good Teaching*. Jossey-Bass, San
Francisco.

Ewan, C. and White, R. (1984). *Teaching Nursing: a Self Instructional
Handbook*. Croom Helm, London.

Flanders, N. (1970). *Analyzing Teacher Behaviour*. Addison-Wesley,
Reading, Massachusetts.

Gallego, A.P. (1983). *Evaluating the School*. Royal College of Nursing,
London.

Gallego, A.P. (1987). Evaluation in nursing education. In *Nursing
Education: Research and Developments*, B. Davis (Ed.), pp 205–35.
Croom Helm, London.

Jeffers, J.M. and Guthrie, D.W. (1988). Self-assessment via video-taping
to maximize teaching effectiveness. *Journal of Continuing Education in
Nursing*, **19(5)**, 223–6.

Lattimer, V.A. and Lattimer, M.G. (1989). *Cluster Centred Practice*.
(Unpublished.)

Mann, F. and Likert, R. (1977). The need for research on the
communication of research results. In *Readings in Evaluation Research*.
Second edition. F.G. Caro (Ed.), pp 125–34. Russell Sage Foundation,
New York.

Mogan, J. and Knox, J.E. (1987). Characteristics of 'best' and 'worst'
clinical teachers as perceived by university nursing faculty and students.
Journal of Advanced Nursing, **12(3)**, 331–7.

Murphy, R. and Torrance, H. (1987). Introduction – towards better
schools? In *Evaluating Education: Issues and Methods*, R. Murphy and
H. Torrance (Eds), pp ix–xiii Harper and Row, London.

Pacini, C.M. and Westphal, C.G. (1988). Evaluating the quality of
education-practice relationships. *Nursing Clinics of North America*, **23(3)**,
671–7.

Parlett, M. and Hamilton, D. (1987). Evaluation as illumination: a new
approach to the study of innovatory programs. In *Evaluating Education:
Issues and Methods*, R. Murphy and H. Torrance (Eds), pp 57–73. Harper
and Row, London.

Sampson, E.E. and Marthas, M.S. (1977). *Group Process for the Health
Professions*. Wiley, Chichester.

Stenhouse, L. (1987). The study of samples and the study of cases. In
Evaluating Education: Issues and Methods, R. Murphy and H. Torrance
(Eds.), pp 74–80. Harper and Row, London.

Stronach, I. (1987). Practical evaluation. In *Evaluating Education: Issues
and Methods*, R. Murphy and H. Torrance (Eds), pp 204–11. Harper
and Row, London.

United Kingdom Central Council for Nursing, Midwifery and Health
Visiting (1989). *Exercising Accountability*. UKCC, London.

Van Ort, S. *et al.* (1986). Developing and implementing a model for
evaluating teaching effectiveness. *Image: Journal of Nursing Scholarship*,
18(3), 114–17.

Walker, R. (1987). Techniques for research. In *Evaluating Education: Issues*

and Methods, R. Murphy and H. Torrance (Eds), pp 225–48. Harper
and Row, London.
Wolf, R.M.   (1979).   *Evaluation in Education: Foundations of Competency
Assessment and Program Review*. Praeger, New York.
Wood, V. and Matthewman, J.   (1987).   Performance of nursing instructors:
an examination of four tools. *Nurse Education Today*, **8(3)**, 131–9.
Zander, A.   (1982).   *Making Groups Effective*. Jossey-Bass, San Francisco.
Zimmerman, L. and Westfall, J.   (1988).   The development and validation
of a scale measuring effective clinical teaching behaviours. *Journal of
Nursing Education*, **27(6)**, 274–7.

Bibliography

Greaves, F.   (1987).   *The Nursing Curriculum: Theory and Practice*. Croom
Helm, London.
Hammersley, M. (Ed.)   (1986).   *Controversies in Classroom Research*. Open
University Press, Milton Keynes.
Handy, C.B.   (1985).   *Understanding Organizations*. Third edition. Penguin,
Harmondsworth.

9 Information Technology: innovation in the curriculum

Keiron Spires

Information Technology (IT) is becoming part of our everyday lives, and is increasingly found in hospitals, GP practices and other care settings. This chapter explores the need for nurses to learn the skills associated with IT and how these skills can be incorporated into nursing curricula.

Why teach computer skills to nurses?

Project 2000 emphasises the need for nurses to be able to analyse critically and be flexible in their approach to nursing. Part of being a professional is the ability to adapt to change and adopt new ideas. As computers are undoubtedly part of today's society and increasingly evident in nursing, nurses cannot abrogate their professional responsibility of exploring the potential of such technology in administration, clinical practice and education (Koch and Rankin, 1987).

Nursing is becoming more complex and more expensive. Accurate, complete and up to date records are required to meet professional, educational, and legal needs, but nurses cannot always afford the time required to assemble records. Also, much of the nursing workload is determined by the medical care prescribed and, although nurses do not initiate this workload, they are required to have staff available in the correct numbers, with the appropriate skiils to meet it and to cope with the inevitable variations in the workload. This requires ways of evaluating whether the care given was appropriate. Technology may be able to help (Scholes *et al.*, 1983).

Nurses functioning as professional carers have every right to expect information technology (IT) to relieve them of routine paperwork. By storing data to be instantly available a computerised patient care information system can take away some of the pressure the increased volume and complexity of records brings. With the acceptance of the Körner reports nurses are expected to be far more accountable and to supply up to date and accurate information both clinically and managerially. The Körner initiative is the first concerted effort to collate computerised data throughout the National Health Service (NHS), the aim being to establish information systems which identify the costs of treating defined groups of patients, so that doctors and nurses can monitor their own performance more effectively. This has led to most Health Authorities computerising information relating to patient administration, as well as personnel, finance and support functions. Nursing, as the biggest budget and manpower sector in hospitals, must surely follow (Fletcher, 1982).

In summary, there will be a need for nurses to adapt to these and other changes, in order to master the increasing complexity of nursing and the complexity of information gathering. It is, therefore, important that nurses explore the issues surrounding computers in nursing.

Computers have been encircled by an aura of technology, hearsay and misinformation which has made a number of people, including many nurses, dismiss them as an intrusion and threat. Such attitudes can be overcome partly by increasing nurses' confidence through education and training, and also by helping them realise that the increased use of computers will allow nurses to enhance their professionalism as they participate *actively* in future developments. Since it is obvious that computers will become an integral part of the ward environment as time goes on, nurses have a professional responsibility to *influence* these developments. There are, moreover, ethical and legal issues involved as well as professional ones. Nurses have a choice then, of allowing managers to implement computer systems into clinical areas as a *fait accompli*, or being involved in what happens to computers in nursing. Nurses cannot be involved effectively if they have not the skills and knowledge to be active participants.

All nurses should therefore have the opportunity to gain sufficient skills so as to allow them to participate in the introduction of technology, to use what technology is available and, perhaps more importantly, to ensure that technology does no harm to patients or clients.

What should we be teaching nurses?

'The literature abounds with claims that the new technologies, especially computers, are full of versatility, and that they are a solution to almost every educational problem. Consequently, we 'jump on the old bandwagon' and rush out to buy the latest hardware and software without defining why it is being purchased' (Armstrong, 1984). Is Nurse Education really preparing nurses for what they face when they qualify, or is it just 'tinkering' with new technologies? As Edmunds (1985) indicates, if nurses do not have a clear idea of what they want and its feasibility, computer managers will themselves set priorities for nursing and nurse education. In order for nurses to take control of these complex technologies they need to learn about their capabilities and limitations.

An editorial in *Computers in Nursing* (1985) claimed that the major obstacle to increased use of computers in nursing practice was a deficit that occurred earlier, during the pre-registration education of nurses. In most respects this is probably still true. Part of this problem may be that nurse education has not identified the skills and knowledge that nurses require in order to cope with computers in nursing.

Reed (1987) identified four areas in which nurses may come into contact with computers: education, clinical, managerial and research. She also highlighted the sorts of applications being used. In nurse management the use of wordprocessors, databases, modems and spreadsheets is already a familiar feature. In hospitals and in the community, databases and modems are increasingly used in sensitive and sophisticated software aiding care delivery, or in monitoring the quality of care. In research the whole range of applications are used a great deal. In education the use of computer assisted learning (CAL) is slowly increasing and some ideas for the computer training needs of nurses have been put forward. These include 'hands on' experience and software awareness relating, for example, to wordprocessing and spreadsheets; a basic understanding of computer concepts and language; a basic idea of systems analysis and design; some insight into hardware design (Reed, 1987; Hoy, 1987). In addition, as previously mentioned, there is also the need to explore the ethical and legal issues surrounding computers in nursing.

The English National Board for Nursing, Midwifery and Health Visiting (ENB) have encouraged schools and colleges of nursing to develop the resources required to integrate CAL into the curricula (ENB, 1986; 1987a). They have laid down guidelines which have encouraged schools to purchase one specific make of computer, namely the Acorn BBC series of microcomputer (Procter, 1987). However, the ENB's support of the BBC machines for CAL may not meet the training needs outlined above for, although applications software such as Wordprocessing is available for this range of machines, they are not industry standard, and the machines and software are unlikely to be met outside of the school. A further issue relates to the purpose of using these machines. The ENB emphasise the development and use of CAL software but it could be argued that CAL is just another option for teachers and should not be seen as the be all and end all of computers. Although production of good CAL is important, there are two issues which need addressing; first, the ability of the BBC range of machines to support powerful CAL packages, and second, the capability of CAL in meeting the needs of the learners.

It is self-evident that the BBC range will never match the power and versatility of the Personal Computer (PC) class of computer, nor will it have the 'big business' backing and expertise to produce good CAL products. Moreover, although CAL in the classroom will help teach keyboard skills to learners, the real advantages are for the teaching staff and the institution. CAL enhances the range of options for teaching, it frees teacher time and may encourage student-centred learning. It will not, however, develop in the learners the full range of skills required.

What is required is an integrated Information Technology thread which explores all the issues surrounding computers in nursing, and provides training in practical keyboard skills which will enable learners to use computers as tools and give them greater insight into IT in the NHS (Fig. 9.1). This will enable them, as qualified nurses, to be in a

---

COMMON FOUNDATION PROGRAMME

Aims
(a) To explore the underlying principles of computer technology.
(b) To enable understanding of the reasons for the enormous growth in this field over recent years.
(c) To enable the students to carry out basic maintenance and fault finding.
(d) To facilitate the development of practical 'user' skills on a range of hardware and software combinations (this does not include programming).

Content
Computers in society, the microchip, inside the computer, hardware combinations, peripherals, use of a variety of software packages.

BRANCH PROGRAMME

Aims
(a) To explore the issues surrounding computers in nursing from an eclectic view.
(b) To enable the students to gain practical skills in applications in the clinical and ward management fields.
(c) To explore the control of IT resources.
(d) To enable the student to use a problem-solving approach to the implementation of IT in nursing.

Content
Computers in nursing from a variety of perspectives. Computers in the NHS (including Körner and devolved resource management). Computers in the hospital setting (resource organisation, decision-making). Computers in the ward: present and future applications.

Fig. 9.1 Summary of a Project 2000 curriculum thread for Information Technology.

position to influence and control the use of computers in nursing rather than being passive recipients of IT.

How do you get 'IT' into the curriculum?

There is no doubt that introducing IT into the curriculum is a complex process. It is a change involving new ideas and technologies, and requires a large amount of resources in order to be successful. Some authors have said that it is vital to have a clear understanding of the situation before the innovative process begins (Greiner, 1967; Gross *et al.*, 1971). In retrospect it may well be seen that the present use of IT in curricula, although planned for, came about more by a process of accident rather than design. This difference between intentional and deliberate change, and accidental or unintentional movements and shifts is recognised by Bolam (1975) who concedes that this distinction is rarely adhered to in the literature.

The process of change is dynamic and takes place over a period of time. This period of time can be thought of in terms of three stages: before the change takes place; when the change takes place; and after the change has taken place. Hull *et al.* (1973) (cited by Bolam, 1975) call these stages antecedent, interactive and consequent, which are perhaps more descriptive than those used by the ENB (1987b) – pre-innovative, the innovative act and post-innovative.

Antecedent phase

The antecedent phase is characterised by three sytems, the *innovation*, the *change agent* and the *user group* (Bolam, 1975). They exist in a specific *environment*. When looking at the introduction of IT into the curriculum, in terms of change theory, it is important to examine these four factors and how they are related. As with any educational analysis, it is not always possible to place particular activities under the headings set out in the literature.

The *innovation* being introduced is, as mentioned above, the introduction of IT into the curriculum. By this it is intended that all students should have a working knowledge of computers in nursing, and basic keyboard skills by the time they qualify. In addition it is recognised that many of the topics or other threads that appear in curricula may have an IT dimension to them (Fig. 9.2). An IT thread then, needs to be developed for each of the courses being run within an institution of nurse education. Alongside the development of the IT thread there must be an acknowledgement of the need for the resources to put it into action, and the need for teaching staff to be able to support the thread.

The knowledge base behind this innovation can be built up from a variety of sources. There is much literature relating to IT in education although not necessarily nurse education. IT has been a fundamental part of general education for some time, and has certainly been an increasing influence in our daily lives. Most hospitals now rely on IT to a greater extent for most management and personnel functions, and to a lesser extent for nursing and medical records and in pharmacy, pathology and x-ray departments. The degree to which nurses are involved in these developments varies, but within many hospitals nurses

---

Aspects which could be part of Nursing Studies or Professional Practice threads, depending on the curriculum in use.

Why nurses need to learn IT skills
  – arrival of IT on ward areas
  – professional responsibility
  – need to know current IT activities in clinical areas

IT in NHS Management
  – exploration of current and future IT practices in the NHS and in particular within the learner's own Health Authority.

Aspects which could be part of Law, Ethics or Social Sciences threads depending on the curriculum in use.

The law
  – principles of confidentiality
  – Data Protection Act
  – computer theft and fraud

Information gathering
  – relevance of collected information
  – move from retrospective to live analysis
  – Körner

Fig. 9.2.   Information Technology components of other curriculum threads.

are using ward-based computers for bedstates, booking out-patient appointments, admissions and getting pathology reports. Nurse managers may be using the personnel system to gain information about sickness rates, budgeting, and general manpower planning. A number of schools of nursing have allocation systems and some have completely integrated record keeping, allocation and school management systems. There is, therefore, certain to be some nursing knowledge base in most hospitals.

There has been little research into IT in nursing and its effects. Some researchers have attempted to show the advantages of using CAL in nurse education, but with few demonstrable results. It may well be that some of the tutorial staff within an institution planning to bring in these changes may have had some experience with computers either at home or on courses, or via a spouse whose work involves computers. Many institutions have some computer resources already available, and many of the students themselves will have had exposure to IT at school. When planning the IT thread it is important that all these sources of knowledge and expertise are tapped.

Many authors have written about the factors which seem to be important in terms of the success or otherwise of the innovation. The main factors would appear to be the relevance of the change, its magnitude, its compatibility and its costs and benefits. First, the *relevance* of the innovation is important to the user group and may rely to a certain extent upon the users feeling that the innovation has some *relative advantage* over current practice, upon its *competitive strength* against other planned changes or activities requiring scarce resources, and also upon its *feasibility* within the organisation (Rogers and Shoemaker, 1971; Bolam, 1975).

The IT thread could be argued as relevant with the increasing level of IT in nursing and the desire by nurses to control its introduction and expansion within their sphere of influence. In terms of competition and feasibility, it is difficult to argue the case for the expensive resources required to teach large groups of students computer skills (Fig. 9 3) and for the valuable time in study blocks which must be gained by displacing other threads or topics. The urgent need for computer skills does seem to outweigh, to some extent, the potential disadvantages of this innovation but the process of having to negotiate for IT resources, and having to argue the value of IT in the curricula, emphasises that there is always a political side to any innovation. This political process is important for the success of the innovation and should not be ignored, when using the systematic approach to change outlined in this chapter.

Second, all of these factors are in turn affected by the *magnitude* of the innovation. This includes the *scale* of the change (fundamental or superficial), and its *trialability*. These in turn affect the innovation's *communicability* which is itself dependent on its *complexity* and *observability* (Rogers and Shoemaker, 1971; Hoyle, 1972; Hull *et al.*, 1973; cited by Bolam, 1975).

The introduction of IT into curricula is an institution-wide change affecting all pre-registration and post-registration courses, and, to some extent, continuing education and in-service training. It is a major change involving all staff and many resources. Although computers are highly visible objects and easy to demonstrate and advertise, the actual computer skills as well as the theory behind IT is a complex subject. It should be recognised early on that, in order to have IT in the curricula, the tutorial staff will have to have an increased understanding of IT and the knowledge and skills required to support students learning IT skills.

Third, the *compatibility* of the innovation with existing values and

	£PER UNIT	UNITS	£TOTAL
INITIAL COSTS			
50 User Network	1595	1	1595
300MB Hard Disk	2995	1	2995
386K File Server	3500	1	3500
		total	8090
WORKSTATIONS			
Comms. Card	450	21	9450
286K computers	500	21	10500
		total	19950
SOFTWARE			
Wordprocessing	210	1	210
	85	20	1700
Spreadsheet		21	1650
Database		21	2000
		total	5560
OTHER COSTS			
Printer	1700	1	1700
Projector	900	1	900
		total	2600
TOTAL OUTLAY LESS INSTALLATION (as at May 1989)			£36200

Fig. 9.3.   Cost of resources for a computer laboratory (20 students).

practices needs to be considered (Rogers and Shoemaker, 1971). Although the innovation will probably be a new area to most of the tutorial staff and to much of the student population, most will feel the need for these sorts of skills and knowledge, particularly when they become aware of the types of IT development happening in their own ward areas, institutions and hospitals. In an educational sense, the computers would allow an added dimension to the student-centred approach favoured by most institutions. Since what research there has been into computers and nurse education seems to show favourable results in terms of educational practices and student results, this should help to put the innovation into a good light. In some respects the innovation could be seen as a stepping-stone to other changes occurring in nurse education.

Lastly, it is important to look at the *costs and benefits* of an innovation. There are serious financial implications of a change of this nature but the advantages are manifold. Benefits such as a greater control of IT in nursing, the increased prestige of the institution, the ability to give students courses in computers in nursing and the increase in status for computer literate nurses all help to outweigh any costs. It should also be recognised that investment in computer resources will allow the running of courses for people outside the institution, or indeed, outside the NHS. This, to some extent, would help to recoup the investment costs.

It is impossible to separate the innovations from the *user group*, this being the group which is either inventing or adopting an innovation or is being aimed at by a change agent. There are several terms for users in the literature: receiver, client, adopter, target and consumer (Bolam, 1975). The user group in this instance may appear to be the student population, but the tutorial staff are in reality the main target group since students may be obliged to undertake whatever topics are in the curricula, and unfortunately often have no control over the form such studies take (i.e. curriculum planning). So in fact the tutorial staff are the main user group of this innovation.

There are six categories of users who may be found in any organisation (Rogers and Shoemaker. 1971: ENB, 1987b). They are normally represented on a continuum between those who strongly support the change, and those who are firmly against it. It is evident that a person's place on this continuum will depend on the change taking place, and a careful assessment of people's feelings about IT in the curriculum will have to be made.

Hoyle (1975) stresses the importance of the 'head teacher' in an educational setting, as far as innovation is concerned. In any institution of nurse education where innovation of this nature is sought, it should be recognised that the head of the institution has to be instrumental in setting the process of change in action, and in supporting the change agent. As Hoyle and many others make clear, it is the head of the institution who will control the 'organisational health' of the environment. This will be discussed later in this chapter.

In this sense it is likely that the head of the institution will be in the *innovator* category. It would be helpful to the change agent if others amongst the senior tutorial staff also fitted into this category or that of *early adopters*. In most institutions there will be a range of views and feelings and a survey of staff would probably find people to fit each of the categories described by Rogers and Shoemaker (1971). Hopefully most, on balance, would tend toward support for the change rather than being firmly opposed to it.

There are ways of influencing the users in order to shift them along the continuum towards supporting the change. These are outlined by the ENB (1987b) based on the work of Havelock and Huberman. By active involvement in both the formulation and implementation of the innovation users can develop a *sense of ownership* of the innovation. In practice most tutorial staff lack the skills and knowledge to formulate

Introduction

The overall aim of this 5 day course is to enable nurse teachers to become computer literate.

The teaching aims of this course are

- To develop understanding of computer 'jargon' and the way computers work
- To increase knowledge of computer strategies in relation to
  (a) the ENB
  (b) the Health Authority
  (c) the Institution itself
- To enable teachers to develop skills in using the institution's micro-computers for
  (a) CAL
  (b) Word Processing
  (c) Specialist Applications
- To develop teachers' skills in using Health Authority systems
- To enable teachers to realise the implications of the Data Protection Act (1984)

Programme

Monday	am	Introduction to the course
		Introduction to computers: a brief look at what makes a computer work. In particular, how to get information in and out of computers, and how to get computers to do what is required of them.
	pm	Starting up: How to start up the institution's micro-computers, and how to use the CAL packages available.
Tuesday	am	Computer Strategy (ENB): a look at what the ENB suggest schools of nursing should be doing with microcomputers; the principles of CAL. Specialist applications: a chance to use some of the specialist applications software available in the institution:
		Statistics packages
		Journal Indexing systems
		Modem and Bulletin Boards
		Teletext Editor
	pm	Introduction to wordprocessing: Please bring a letter/handout to this session, which will include preparation of work for wordprocessing, and 'hands on' production of a finished piece of work.
Wednesday		Wordprocessing workshop

Thursday   am Data Protection Act: a look at this Act, and in particular its implications for nursing. Introduction to Health Authority Computer System(s).

                pm Demonstration of Health Authority System(s).

Friday   am The future for computers in the institution: a discussion on planning for the future, both in terms of equipment and curriculum development.

                pm Evaluation

Fig. 9.4 A five day Information Technology course for nurse teachers

an IT thread, but could be involved in its implementation by being able to influence the thread at curriculum planning meetings and in the organisation of study blocks. They should, moreover, be able to influence the links between the IT thread and the other curriculum threads. There should also be *informal personal contracts* in operation in the form of tutorial staff being taught computer skills informally and formally, individually and in groups. This raising of awareness of IT within the institution could be aided by projects such as the publication of a school newsletter using computer technology; linking the library to Datastar (a large computer in Switzerland allowing computerised library searchers); and using school computers to produce teaching aids (for example overhead projection transparancies) for tutorial staff.

A planned and systematic approach to raising IT awareness could be to run short 'in-house' courses for staff (Fig. 9.4). Other contracts could be initiated by tutorial staff who have a particular need, or the change agent could identify areas where IT could be of help in the institution such as statistical analysis of course results and evaluations.

Opinion leaders need to be involved at an early stage, and could be particularly effective in large formal staff meetings, or in smaller 'team' meetings. Often the senior staff are opinion leaders, but if the organisational health of the institution is such that a democratic environment exists in which the opinions of all staff are thought to be of worth then the opinion leaders will be more diverse. Although many staff are likely to be in favour of introducing IT into the curriculum from the outset, it may well be that some will be against it if the innovation is seen as being a top down change i.e. power-coercive. (This is discussed later in the chapter.) The need for *information and support* should be recognised, and this may mean the appointment of a member of staff with specialist skills in IT. This person is likely to be the change agent and would be responsible for raising awareness of the staff as outlined above, and for supporting those implementing the change or experimenting with IT.

It can be seen that the *change agent* has a major effect both on the users and on the environment in which the change takes place. It is important therefore, that this person has the necessary skills and knowledge in IT and thus has some credibility. The job description of the change agent should include those fundamental functions discussed by the ENB (1987b):

(i)   to diagnose the need;
(ii)   to identify and clarify goals of change;
(iii)   to develop strategies and tactics to introduce change; and
(iv)   to establish and maintain a working relationship with change users.

Although many of these functions may be embedded in the job description of the change agent, they are not likely to be explicit in this way. In discussing the effect of the change agent on the users some of these functions have already been described.

Bolam (1975) suggests that the most important characteristic of the change agent is an *authority relationship* with the users. This could be based on administrative status, professional colleagueship, external consultancy or a combination of the three. The ENB (1987b) point out the value of appointing someone into a 'special' post. They also cite Rogers and Shoemaker (1971) who found that a change agent's success in introducing change was positively related to:

(i)   the extent of the change agent's effort;
(ii)   the change agent's client orientation;
(iii)   the compatability of the innovation (discussed earlier);
(iv)   the change agent's empathy with users;
(v)   the extent to which the change agent worked through opinion leaders (discussed earlier);
(vi)   the change agent's credibility in the eyes of the users; and
(vii)   the change agent's efforts to increase the users' ability to evaluate the innovation.

Some of these areas have been discussed above, others involve the personal characteristics and ability of the change agent.

The innovation, the users and the change agent have been shown to have very close links, and in fact they could be said to be interdependent to some extent. They do not exist in a vacuum but in a specific *environment* which itself influences the other factors and vice versa. Hoyle (1975), citing Miles (1965), discusses the need for good 'organisational health' if an innovation is to succeed. The ENB (1987b) call this being 'ripe for change'. They argue that this involves the co-existence of five conditions. The first of these is *openness* and the second, *interpersonal information linkages*. To be 'ripe for change' an institution should be one in which questioning and critical reflectivity is encouraged. There need to be formal and informal forums in which these expressions can be made and good channels of communication, both vertically and horizontally. There should be an atmosphere in which healthy open discussion and debate can take place. For example, are institutional staff meetings purely information giving, or are staff allowed to air their views, and critically discuss events affecting the institution? Is there any way for staff to meet and debate issues that concern them without the presence of more senior staff inhibiting the discussion? Are 'sanctions' taken against those who speak out? All these areas should be explored and assessed.

The third condition associated with 'ripeness for change' is *freedom from organisational constraints*. To be successful the introduction of IT needs to be encouraged and the results of changes should be freely disseminated. Staff should be encouraged to develop specialist areas like IT, and to take responsibility for them. Even though the institution may have a traditional hierarchy, and specialist teachers may be responsible to senior tutors, personal autonomy should be given to a large extent. Staff should be held accountable for their specialist area, rather than accountability falling to a 'team'.

The fourth condition is *supportive leadership*. The senior staff must be supportive of the innovation if it is to succeed. The head of the institution must be prepared to exercise the necessary power to implement, sustain and institutionalise the innovation as the change agent requires. If the head of the institution or a majority of senior staff are not in favour of the introduction of IT into the curriculum then the focus of the change agent should be on changing these views *before* attempting to introduce the change.

The last condition is *trust*. The atmosphere of the institution should be one of professional collegiality with much collaboration and sharing of ideas and activities. This may be in the form of collaboration in teaching, in writing articles or books and in generally sharing what is going on in teams or specialist areas. It also suggests peer evaluation and a safe and supportive climate for discussion or experimentation within the peer group.

Although the description of the five factors is very idealistic, it is important to assess the institution and its organisational health. It may well be that work is required to improve some of these areas before an innovation such as the introduction of IT into the curriculum is attempted.

As well as assessing the state of organisational health it is necessary to look for the existence of barriers to change within the environment. The two main areas to examine are personal resistance to change and organisational barriers. These probably exist in all institutions to a greater or lesser degree and an important part of the antecedent phase is the breaking down of these barriers.

The personal resistance to change is a response to the anxiety that change evokes and is entirely normal. It can be overcome in many ways – most of which have already been mentioned. Fullan (1982) mentions three factors at work in this situation. First he emphasises that change is *multidimensional* in that it is associated with the use of new materials or technologies, new teaching approaches and a change in educational beliefs. Change can vary according to these dimensions within an individual as well as within a group. Second, Fullan suggests that bringing about change involves people's occupational identity, their sense of competence, and their self-concept. In particular he stresses that 'the need and difficulty for individuals to develop a sense of meaning about change is manifest'. Third, is the fact that change consists of a *dynamic inter-relationship* of the various dimensions. For example, the effective use of educational materials depends on how they articulate with people's educational beliefs and teaching approaches. Fullan believes that 'whether or not people develop meaning in relation to these aspects is fundamentally the problem'. This highlights the fact that the use of a systematic approach to change must also take account of these factors if a successful innovation is to take place.

ENB (1987b) suggested that organisational barriers include:
— lack of understanding by the intended users as to how the change will effect their role, relationships and practices;
— a lack of in-service training;
— inadequate resource allocation (time, people, money, materials);
— lack of managerial and/or political support within an authority; and
— too many competing innovations being introduced at the same time.

Some of these are bound to be present in any institution of nurse education. The role of the tutorial staff may change, and this needs to be recognised by both the change agent and the user group. For example, the need to support students who are learning computer skills may require tutorial staff to obtain sufficient knowledge and skills to be able to do this.

In-service training will need to be provided and an ongoing programme of training instituted (Fig. 9.4). The question of resources is a thorny one. As previously stated, IT resources are expensive. There is no doubt that the ideal resources would be a computer 'laboratory' with the equipment discussed earlier. The small amount of resources currently available in most institutions would definitely slow down such an innovation. There are also, at present, many other changes taking place in nurse education, ranging from massive changes in curricula for Project 2000, to changes in teaching styles and the preparation of nurse teachers themselves. All these changes result in at least a temporary increase in staff workloads. Time is therefore likely to be a scarce resource.

The three factors of innovation, user group and change agent have been shown to be closely linked, though they remain separate until innovation begins. All of these factors are capable of being assessed, and innovation should be easier if it is brought about in a planned and systematic way taking all the factors into account.

Interactive phase

The interactive phase, during which interaction between the factors takes place, is the most critical and the most complex as far as the outcome of the innovation is concerned. The interactive phase begins during the dissemination or awareness stage and is certainly taking place during the trial and implementation stages. Key questions here relate to the change agent's strategies and communication. Bolam (1975) summarises three strategies discussed in Bennis *et al.* (1969):

Power-coercive strategies depend upon access to political, legal, administrative and economic resources. Typically they involve the use of legal or administrative power

Normative-Re-educative strategies assume that effective innovation requires a change of attitudes, relationships, values and skills and therefore, the activation of forces within the client system (user group) .

Empirical-rational strategies assume that (people) are reasonable and will respond best to rational explanation and demonstration. Typically they involve the use of education, training and publications to disseminate knowledge and research findings.

From the discussion on the factors in the antecedent phase, elements of all three strategies are likely to be used.

The involvement of the head of the institution, particularly if a person is appointed to a special IT post, is in part power-coercive. In fact power-coercive strategies are at work from outside the institution. The ENB has already put out documents outlining their intentions in the area of IT.

By raising the awareness of tutorial staff towards IT and its uses, and in particular by trying to make IT useful to them, values can be changed and new skills gained. By making IT useful to tutorial staff they will be encouraged to learn more and to pass on their experience to others. Certainly, running in-house courses and individual training sessions will do much to reduce any fears and anxieties about IT, and staff can be involved in discussions about the introduction of the IT thread into the curriculum. These are all normative-re-educative strategies.

Running courses and training sessions could also be said to be a rational-empirical strategy, as is the dissemination of information by using IT, and any other 'advertising ploys' available. This enables teachers to see for themselves the importance of the innovation in the light of current trends in nursing.

Most authors writing about change theory accept this combination of approaches and indeed a fourth strategy has been put forward that combines and co-ordinates the elements that exist in all of them (Sieber, 1971; cited by Ketefian, 1978).

Consequent phase

There should be an ongoing evaluation of the process of change throughout, and even when still planning the first two phases of the introduction of IT into the curricula it is important to look forward to the third or consequent phase. After the interactive process is complete and implementation of the innovation is finished, the three factors discussed above will, to some extent, separate out again (Bolam, 1975). It will be possible then to assess each of the factors, as was done in the antecedent phase, to see what, if any, differences there are. Teaching methods may have changed, opinions and values will almost certainly have changed. Bolam (1975) suggests that the change agent may have learned some new techniques in the management of change! The innovation may have undergone change or been revised by the user group.

Bolam (1975) describes several ways the user group may respond during the interactive and consequent stages. For example, the user group may *reject* or *resist* the innovation. One variant of resistance is the 'façade phenomenon' in which staff may unintentionally 'put on a front' that suggests the innovation is working well, even though 'objective' outsiders would disagree (Smith and Keith, 1971; cited by Bolam, 1975). The users may *adapt* the innovation, even to the degree where it bears no relation to the innovation the change agent was originally seeking. The innovation may become fully *institutionalised* and an enthusiastic user group may become *advocates* of IT!

At a time of challenge and opportunity in nurse education, those teachers who are considering developing the Information Technology component of their curricula may gain inspiration from Armstrong (1984) who suggests that

'as we strive for excellence, the decision for using alternative strategies is ours – either lift the anchor or maintain the status quo. If you decide to take the plunge . . .
Study all alternative methods,
Chart your course, but don't expect smooth sailing.
Batten down the hatches.
Use all relevant navigational aids.
Steady at the helm . . .
Damn the torpedoes . . .
And full speed ahead.'

(Hutchinson, 1976; cited by Armstrong, 1984)

References

Armstrong, M.L. (1984). Riding the waves with the new technologies. *Journal of Continuing Education in Nursing*, **15(5)**, 152–3.

Bolam, R. (1975). The management of educational change: towards a conceptual framework. In *Curriculum Innovation*, A. Harris *et al.* (Eds), pp 273–90. Croom Helm, London.

Computers in Nursing (1985). Editorial. *Computers in Nursing* **4(3)**, 102, 136.

Edmunds, L. (1985). Hospital information systems for nursing problems and possibilities. *Proceedings of the 9th Annual Symposium on Computer Applications in Medical Care*, pp 785–9. Institute of Electrical and Electronics Engineers Computer Society Press, Washington, D.C.

English National Board for Nursing, Midwifery and Health Visiting (1986). *A Framework for the Development of Computer Assisted Learning (CAL) for Nurses, Midwives and Health Visitors: Draft*. ENB, London.

English National Board for Nursing, Midwifery and Health Visiting (1987a). *A Framework for the Development of Computer Assisted Learning (CAL) for Nurses, Midwives and Health Visitors: Revised Report*. ENB, London.

English National Board for Nursing, Midwifery and Health Visiting (1987b). *Managing Change in Nursing Education – Section 3: The Process of Innovation*. ENB, London.

Fletcher, S. (1982). Körner report: bridging the information gap. *Health and Social Service Journal*, **92(4821)**, 1315–17.

Fullan, M. (1982). *The Meaning of Educational Change*. OISE Press/Ontario Institute for Studies in Education, Toronto.

Greiner, L.E. (1967). Antecedents of planned organisational change. *Journal of Applied Behavioural Science*, **3(1)**, 51–85.

Gross, N. *et al.* (1971). *Implementing Organisational Innovations*. Harper and Row, London.

Hoy, R. (1987). The computer – an aid to nursing care. *Senior Nurse*, **7(3)**, 22–3.

Hoyle, E. (1975). Planned organizational change in education. In *Curriculum Innovation*, A. Harris *et al.* (Eds), pp 291–311. Croom Helm, London.

Ketefian, S. (1978). Strategies of curriculum change. *International Nursing Review*, **25(1)**, 14–21, 24.

Koch, B. and Rankin, J. (Eds) (1987). *Computers and Their Applications in Nursing*. Harper and Row, London.

Procter, P. (1987). CAL: the ENB approach. *Senior Nurse*, **7(5)**, 48.

Reed, V. (1987). New nursing horizons in information technology. *Senior Nurse*, **7(3)**, 19–21.

Rogers, E.M. and Shoemaker, F.F. (1971). *Communication of Innovations: a Cross-Cultural Approach*. Collier-Macmillan, London.

Scholes, M. *et al.* (Eds) (1983). *The Impact of Computers on Nursing: an International Review*. Elsevier Science, Amsterdam.

10 Improving curriculum decision-making

Stella Pendleton

'There's too much emphasis on what students can *do*. What about how they're developing as people?'

'Students get their heads stuffed full of highbrow knowledge and then they can't even take a blood pressure properly.'

'All this about students choosing what they want to do. We'll never cover everything they need to know.'

'I feel a bit uneasy about political and social issues being part of the curriculum. The students probably know more than I do about some of these things.'

The above comments might be stated openly in a curriculum develop-ment group meeting or be expressed privately to like-minded colleagues. They might remain as unspoken thoughts. Nevertheless, they capture some of the contradictions embedded in the four ideologies discussed in Chapter one: instrumentalism, liberal humanism, progressivism and reconstructionism. Yet issues relating to the nature of nursing education and control of teaching and learning processes and outcomes need to be examined as part of the curriculum process, and an attempt made to draw on the best of all the ideologies in order to achieve balance in the curriculum.

The question of choosing from alternatives and achieving balance is, however, problematic. The behavioural objectives model suggests a rational and orderly set of procedures for planning a curriculum: state your purposes in terms of aims and objectives, select and organise content and learning experiences as the means by which students will achieve the objectives, and then evaluate to find out whether the objec-tives have been achieved. Yet Tyler (1949), whose work has been so influential in the behavioural objectives movement, stated that his book was 'not a manual for curriculum construction' but simply outlined 'one way of viewing an instructional program'. In spite of this the behavioural objectives model came to be seen as a blueprint for curriculum development (Sockett, 1976), and the process ignored, as Tyler had done, the problems of choosing and achieving consensus about objectives (Reid, 1975). It is suggested here, however, that differences in ideologies need to be faced and indeed exploited as a way of improving curriculum decision-making. The idea of blueprints for curriculum construction is also suspect since it suggests that curricula are designed by standard teachers, for standard students, in standard settings. Yet the curriculum is planned and enacted by particular groups of teachers for and with specific students, in unique settings. Some general constraints will be shared with other schools but these will never be exactly the same for individual institutions. The notion of curriculum planning as an orderly sequence of procedures also seems somewhat removed from everyday reality where the process often seems exploratory and rather messy. The fact is that the behavioural objectives model is prescriptive rather than descriptive, that is, it suggests how curricula *should* be planned, rather than describing how they actually *are* planned. Prescriptive models are no doubt used by some as a framework for writing curriculum documents but they are arguably of limited value in the planning process. In order to explore this further, it is necessary to consider the nature of curriculum problems.

The nature of curriculum problems

Reid (1978) suggests that effective curricular practice relates to effective decision-making, which is in turn a kind of problem-solving. He asserts that how we view curriculum problems will determine the theoretical stance we adopt in trying to solve them, and he describes two basic categories of problems: theoretic and practical. Theoretic problems can be translated into questions requiring description or explanation as answers. 'What have the new set of students had on nursing theory?' and 'How do adults learn?' are examples of theoretic questions. Practical problems, on the other hand, relate to questions about what to do or how to do it. Some of these problems are procedural, that is, they can be tackled by applying known procedures. 'How do I work the film projector?' is an example of a practical procedural problem. Reid (1978) suggests that those who advocate planning by behavioural objectives would say that curriculum problems were practical procedural problems: they are problems which can be solved by applying an appropriate technique. However, Reid (1978) suggests that most curriculum problems, like many everyday problems, are *uncertain* practical problems, and that they relate to questions about *what* students should learn and *how* curricular decisions should be taken and implemented. When these problems involve words like 'ought' they have moral and ethical implications. 'How ought we to formulate the school's philosophy?' is an example of an uncertain practical problem, with ethical implications. Reid (1978) describes the features of uncertain practical problems:

1. They involve questions that have to be answered even if the answer is to do nothing.
2. The grounds on which decisions have to be made are uncertain.
3. Decisions have to be taken in the context of past events and the current situation.
4. Each problem occurs at a particular time and in a specific context and so is unique.
5. Problems involve choosing between conflicting aims and values.
6. The outcome will always be to some degree unpredictable.
7. The justification of an action does not lie in the act itself but in the ends we intend to achieve by it.

Such problems are tackled not by applying set procedures or rules but by 'practical reasoning' (Reid, 1978). The problem 'How ought we to formulate the school's philosophy?' is characterised by the seven features. It requires an answer but there are no infallible rules to help decide whose interests and arguments should hold sway. The decision is not taken in a vacuum: the school's traditions and current arrangements, such as staff structures, all have a bearing on the problem, to say nothing of the personalities and groupings of the staff themselves. Conflicting values and aims are involved not only in agreeing philosophical statements but in deciding who ought to participate in discussions. We might want to include all the qualified staff involved with students in school and practice settings, but to meet various deadlines the philosophy might have to be formulated by a representative core group. The outcome cannot be predicted with certainty. The process of formulating the philosophy and the actual philosophical statement may not be what we expected, and there may be unexpected repercussions from staff who felt excluded. Finally, the goal of our solution is not to formulate a philosophy but to try to provide the best educational experience for our students and the highest standard of care for clients and patients. That is our justification for the philosophical statement formulated.

Reid (1978) suggests that sometimes solving a practical problem may involve a mixture of modes. Thus in the above example a procedural element could be introduced by using the Gibson technique mentioned in Chapter 1. However, the outcome would still be uncertain as one could not predict how participants would respond to and adapt the statements on the cards. In summary Reid (1978) contends that 'problems are uncertain when the grounds for decision are unclear, when there are conflicts of aims, when the problems relate to unique contexts, when other people with varying wants and desires are affected by the solutions to them – any one or more of these features points to the existence of an uncertain problem'. Answering practical problems may involve a consideration of theoretic problems, but it is in the context of the 'practical' (what and how to do) that curriculum problems are raised (Reid, 1978). The relationship between the theoretic and the practical is a key concern of Schwab (1969) for he, like Reid, sees curriculum problems as belonging to the realm of the 'practical'. Schwab describes various 'arts' of curriculum planning.

Curriculum arts

Schwab (1969) asserts that theories deal with the general, whereas curriculum is concerned with the particular: with specific students, teachers and settings. Moreover, individual educational theories only give a partial view, stressing for example social need or change, or the individual or structures of knowledge. Yet in practice, Schwab (1969) argues, these theories constitute one complex, organic unity. Schwab (1971;1983) describes various intermingling arts used to reconcile the incongruities between theory and practice. For example, the *practical arts* include arts of perception which would help a nurse teacher to see not a theoretical, archetypal 'adult learner' but Mary Brown who is anxious about coping with the course and is trying to do so with her husband, three children and two dogs to look after. Other practical arts involve formulating curriculum problems in different ways; weighing up and choosing from the alternative formulations; generating alternative possible solutions; thinking through and rehearsing their possible consequences; weighing up and choosing solutions; deciding when to act.

The related *eclectic arts* are concerned with selecting from different theories, adjusting them and perhaps combining a number of incomplete views. Selecting and adapting the best elements from the four ideologies discussed in Chapter 1 would be an example of the eclectic arts, provided the selection involved understanding and judgement. Chapter 2 provides a worked example of how the eclectic arts could be used to plan the ethics component of a curriculum in nursing education. It should be noted that the 'eclectic curriculum' described by Beattie (1987) lacks rigour and would not be an example of Schwab's eclectic arts. The dialectical curriculum advocated by Beattie (1987) would, however, involve the eclectic arts, for it requires purposeful and principled planners, committed to understanding different approaches to the curriculum, unmasking underlying assumptions, combining different approaches and creating new coalitions, which in turn will eventually break down. Beattie's (1987) dialectical curriculum has the characteristics of what Schwab (1969) calls a 'sound eclectic', that is, it allows for '*changing* connections and *differing* orderings at different times of these separate theories ...'

'The practical' then, for Schwab (1969), is 'a discipline concerned with choice and action, in contrast with the theoretic which is concerned with knowledge'. The 'arts' are so termed because they cannot be reduced to rules, but rather require modification and adjustment according to differing circumstances (Schwab, 1971). Schwab places much emphasis on the composition and functioning of curriculum development groups.

Curriculum development groups

Schwab (1973) suggests that four elements of education (or 'commonplaces') must be represented on the curriculum group. Two or more commonplaces, however, may be represented by one person. First, there must be someone familiar with the *subject matter* under discussion. Second, there should be someone who understands the difficulties, anxieties and aspirations of *students*. Third, the *milieux* should be represented. In nursing education this could include lay and nursing representatives from the community and other practice settings; those who are familiar with the requirements of professional and academic bodies, the availability of resources including the library, and the general authority structure of the school. Fourth, the *teachers* should be represented so that, for example, any staff development needs required by curriculum change could be highlighted. Schwab also recommends a *curriculum specialist* who should co-ordinate the commonplaces, ensuring an appropriate emphasis among them, and maintaining a deliberative mode of discussion, in which 'all pool their ingenuities, insights, and perceptions in the interest of discovering the most promising possibilities for trial, rather than forming sides, each of which look only to the strengths of one selected alternative . . .' (Schwab, 1983).

The process of deliberation is spiral and can involve skipping back and forth between the different stages involved in tackling the problem. Roby (1986) calls this 'backtracking'. 'Critical reflection' helps ensure there is no inappropriate bias towards any of the commonplaces and that a range of problem formulations and solutions are considered (Roby, 1986). Roby also suggests that the group's deliberative responsibilities include review and revision of the actions implemented.

Curriculum planning then, for Schwab, involves a group of people representing the main bodies of experience relating to education. Using the eclectic arts involves drawing on a range of general theories, adapting them to the particular instance in hand. The practical arts require representatives of the commonplaces to consider a wide range of alternatives in all the stages of problem appreciation, formulation and solution (Fig. 10.1). It involves what Reid (1981) calls a spirit of 'critical pluralism' and would mean that a curriculum's design was specified by the series of decisions that produced it (Walker, 1971). Key words in this approach are 'deliberation', 'argument', 'judgement', 'justification' and 'action' (Reid, 1978) rather than 'rules' and 'procedures'. It is in this light that the contributions in this book should be viewed: not as

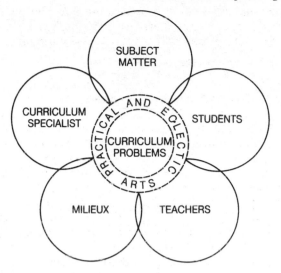

Fig. 10.1 Curriculum planning using the practical and eclectic arts (derived from Schwab, 1973).

prescriptions for action but as ideas to be reflected upon and adapted to suit unique situations.

Nursing education is going through a period of great change which can open up rich possibilities for choice and action. We need nurses with a sound knowledge base who can deliver competent and sensitive care, but we must also foster questing, critical spirits who are able to push back the frontiers of knowledge and see new possibilities for nursing in the creation of a better society. It is hoped that this book will be a contribution both to educational developments related to Project 2000, and to the wider aspirations of Health for All by the year 2000. For as Hellberg (1988) argues, 'No one is fully healthy as long as some of us are sick, suffering and dying from causes that could have been prevented.'

References

Beattie, A. (1987). Making a curriculum work. In *The Curriculum in Nursing Education*, P. Allan and M. Jolley (Eds), pp 15–34. Croom Helm, London.

Hellberg, H. (1988). An evolving process. *World Health*, Jan./Feb., 5–9.

Reid, W.A. (1975). The changing curriculum: theory and practice. In *Case Studies in Curriculum Change. Great Britain and the United States*, W.A. Reid and D.F. Walker (Eds), pp 240–59. Routledge and Kegan Paul, London.

Reid, W.A.   (1978).   *Thinking about the Curriculum. The Nature and Treatment of Curriculum Problems.* Routledge and Kegan Paul, London.

Reid, W.A.   (1981).   The deliberative approach to the study of the curriculum and its relation to critical pluralism. In *Rethinking Curriculum Studies*, M. Lawn and L. Barton (Eds), pp 160–87. Croom Helm, London.

Roby, T.W.   (1986).   Habits impeding deliberation. In *Recent Developments in Curriculum Studies*, P.H. Taylor (Ed.), pp 41–69. NFER – Nelson, Windsor.

Schwab, J.J.   (1969).   The practical: a language for curriculum. *School Review*, **78**, Nov., 1–23.

Schwab, J.J.   (1971).   The practical: arts of eclectic. *School Review*, **79**, Aug., 493–542.

Schwab, J.J.,   (1973).   The practical 3: translation into curriculum. *School Review*, **81**, Aug., 501–22.

Schwab, J.J.   (1983).   The practical 4: something for curriculum professors to do. *Curriculum Inquiry*, **13(3)**, 239–65.

Sockett, H.   (1976).   *Designing the Curriculum.* Open Books, London.

Tyler, R.W.   (1949).   *Basic Principles of Curriculum and Instruction.* University of Chicago Press, Chicago.

Walker, D.F.   (1971).   A naturalistic model for curriculum development. *School Review*, **80**, Nov., 51–65.

Index